an
intimate life

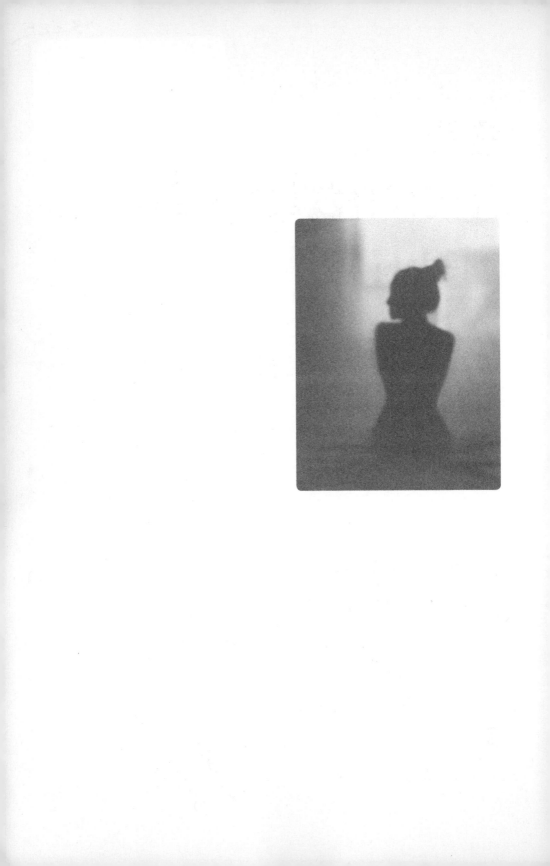

an
intimate life
sex, love, and my journey as a surrogate partner

cheryl t. cohen greene

with lorna garano

SOFT SKULL PRESS
AN IMPRINT OF COUNTERPOINT

a note on names and other identifying details

Throughout this book I share stories from my practice. Names, physical charac-
teristics, and mannerisms have been changed to secure the privacy of my clients.
Many of the client stories presented here occurred many years ago, and, because
of that, I have had to reconstruct dialogue and sensory details that have escaped
memory. In addition, to protect their privacy, I have given pseudonyms to many
of my personal friends, family members, and acquaintances.

Copyright © 2012 by Cheryl T. Cohen Greene with Lorna Garano

Library of Congress Cataloging-in Publication is available.
ISBN 978-1-59376-506-4

Cover design by Natalya Bolnova
Interior design by Elyse Strongin, Neuwirth & Associates, Inc.

Soft Skull Press
An Imprint of COUNTERPOINT
1919 Fifth Street
Berkeley, CA 94710
www.softskull.com

Printed in the United States of America
Distributed by Publishers Group West

10 9 8 7 6 5 4 3 2 1

For my husband, Bob,
whose love and support made this book possible.
I love you!

contents

foreword

Surrogate partner therapy involves three people: the client, the surrogate partner, and the "talk" therapist who weaves it all together. That's me. I make the initial recommendation to incorporate surrogate partner therapy for selected clients.

Once the process has started, the surrogate partner and I confer after each surrogate/client meeting and plan the next. Then the client processes the surrogate experience in a "talk" therapy appointment with me. Cheryl and I have talked through more than one hundred sexual journeys of clients seeking something better.

Thirty years of collaborating about clients with Cheryl has taught me many things. Here are three of the most important: Sex therapy, like life, is never linear, so keeping a spare tank of energy around is always a good strategy. An open-hearted surrogate partner can find real sexual attractiveness in a person least likely to grace the cover of a magazine. And last, the Age of AIDS won't stop a brilliant surrogate partner from doing her work.

Cheryl is one of a kind. She's the person I want to sit next to at sexuality conferences to get her unique take on the research and what it means to her work. She readily generates a no-punches-pulled sexual realism, but it's wrapped in a soft blanket of optimism and nearly boundless compassion.

She *has* to be compassionate. Genuine empathy is required when talking honestly with another naked person about how to touch and receive touch. It's also a necessity when explaining the crucial importance of adopting good sexual hygiene for future sexual partners. A surrogate partner can't be role-modeling sexual communication that works in the real world if it's insincere. Sitting naked face-to-face, eyes-to-eyes for all these years has fostered an unconventional yet very rewarding career for Cheryl.

Surrogate partners are educators for their clients and they are "normalizers." Many clients enter sex therapy with a near-terminal case of uniqueness, thinking that they are beyond help and hope. Many clients whom I've referred to Cheryl came into my practice with the mental equivalent of "one shoe nailed down to the floor." They kept circling around and around their "stuff," unable to change—and felt stuck with their sexual problems. And while surrogate therapy is centered around the client, it's also very much about leading the client out of the set of ideas that nailed the shoe down in the first place.

Clients aren't the only ones with set ideas about sex. I recall attending a sexuality conference at which Cheryl was presenting. It was 1985; AIDS was a reality in the world of sexual contact. The audience of sex therapists, researchers, and educators sat in the audience eagerly awaiting Cheryl's presentation on being a surrogate partner when serious, life-threatening, sexually communicable conditions had entered the landscape. How could a surrogate possibly use a condom with a man with erection dysfunction?

Like most conferences in hotels, there was a table at the back of the room with a continental breakfast. As Cheryl got to the condom part of her presentation, she asked for someone in the audience to get her a banana from the table. Chuckles rippled through the room. Once the banana fetcher had volunteered, Cheryl asked him to eat the banana—more chuckles.

Then Cheryl asked the banana eater to bring her the peel. There, before a convention room full of people, Cheryl opened a condom packet and, holding the peel in one hand, slipped the condom over it in about three seconds. The resemblance between the empty banana peel and a flaccid penis was unmistakable. Case closed.

Many clients doubt their sexual attractiveness. I remember asking Cheryl how she was doing with one particular man I had referred to her. We both knew that a part of his sexual growth would involve his believing that a woman could be turned on by him. I asked her how she was working with that part of it. She replied instantly with her distinct Boston accent, "Oh, he has really great ears and a great neck. I find them sexy." And that's why the amazing story of Mark, in the opening chapter, rings so true. If anyone had a reason to wonder about his attractiveness, it was Mark.

One would think that after doing this work for so many years, Cheryl would become slightly jaded about her clients or blasé about teaching some of the same concepts over and over. But she doesn't. Each time we confer about a recent session with our mutual client, there's Cheryl explaining in detail exactly what she said to the client— as if it was the first time I had heard it or that she had said it. There is no way to pretend such freshness, but it's the reason why a woman nearly 70 years of age can do the work she does with such joy and such purpose.

We have shared the lectern at conferences, witnessed major passages in each other's lives, and stepped into various media settings together hoping to enlighten—only to find the wizardry of video edits sometimes negating our educational intentions. I am honored to write the Foreword for a book that reads like a cliff-hanger despite the fact that I know all the twists and turns of the plot, many of the characters, and how it all turns out. I hope that you will find it, as I have, a privilege to listen in on her thoughts.

—Louanne Cole Weston, Ph.D.

introduction

I have had over nine hundred sex partners. I haven't had intercourse with all of them, but I've had it with most of them. I sometimes reveal this in the talks I give, and, as you can imagine, it sparks a strong reaction. Often, I ask the audience what words come to mind when they hear this figure. Here are a few of the most common: whore, skank, slut. Well, I'm none of those—even though some people will undoubtedly disagree. I am a surrogate partner. These days, people hear that title and think what I do involves carrying children for infertile couples. When I explain to them that I use hands-on methods to help clients overcome sexual difficulties, they come away only slightly less confused. Isn't that prostitution? they wonder, sometimes aloud.

Whereas prostitution is one of the world's oldest professions, surrogacy is one of the newest. Clients are always referred to me by talk-therapist colleagues. They may be suffering from erectile dysfunction, premature ejaculation, anxiety around their sexuality, little or no sexual experience, difficulty communicating, poor body image, or various combinations of these issues. Virtually all of the men (and sometimes women) I see long for more intimate and loving relationships in and out of the bedroom. The work of a surrogate is to give them the essential tools for building healthy and loving relationships.

As a surrogate, I have a series of exercises I use with clients to help them resolve problems and achieve their goals. A good deal of my time is also spent educating them about anatomy and sexuality. I work closely with the referring therapist, checking in with him or her after each session to discuss the client's progress. Clients typically see me for six to eight sessions. One of the biggest misconceptions about surrogacy work is how much intercourse takes place during those sessions. It's true that I have sex with most of my clients, but it is only after we have gone through a number of exercises designed to develop body awareness, address body image issues, achieve relaxation, and hone communication skills. It is usually in the later sessions that we have sex. It's worth noting that I am a "surrogate partner," not a "sex surrogate." My ultimate aim is to model a healthy intimate relationship for a client, and that involves much more than intercourse.

My clients come from all races and socioeconomic backgrounds. The youngest client I worked with was eighteen and the oldest was eighty-nine. They are CEOs, truck drivers, attorneys, and carpenters. Some are hunks; others are average looking. I've worked with a virgin septuagenarian, a college student suffering from premature ejaculation, and men of all ages who don't know how to communicate about sex.

℘

I started this work in 1973, and my journey to it spans our society's sexual revolution and my own. I grew up in the '40s and '50s, a time when sex education was—to put it mildly—lacking. As I educated myself, I found that most of what I had been taught about sex was distorted or wrong. The lessons came from the playground, the church, and the media. My parents could barely talk about sex, much less inform me about it. Unfortunately, many parents today remain as ill-equipped to provide reliable, nonjudgmental sex education as mine were a half a century ago. I often think about how much smarter, healthier, and happier our kids would be if parents had the information and skills to have honest, age-appropriate discussions with them.

Despite what I and many others had hoped for in the exhilarating days of the sexual revolution, too many of us remain mystified about sex and about our bodies. The assault on fact-based sex education led by those who wish to turn back the clock, and the barrage of misinformation we get from the twenty-four-hour media cycle, have many of us as confused as ever. We joke about sex, rail against sex, expose people for having inappropriate sex, and, although I'm hardly the first one to point it out, use sex to sell everything from chewing gum to SUVs. What we have real trouble with, however, is having an honest, mature, and nonjudgmental public conversation about it.

I have wanted to tell my story for a long time, and my motivation for this has evolved and expanded over the years. One thing that has not changed is my belief in the power of stories to inspire and challenge us. My life is, in many ways, a paradigmatic one. I grew up during a time in which rigid dogma about women's sexuality held sway. It came from both religious and secular sources. When I look back on my life, I marvel at how it conferred so much shame and guilt around one of the most natural and healthy human impulses, and at the impact that had on me as a young person. But, I am a baby boomer. My young life straddled two eras. I was in my twenties in the 1960s. The shifting social winds of the time encouraged me to question and rethink nearly everything I had been taught. Held up to daylight, many of the beliefs about sexuality that I had been inculcated with as a child didn't survive. This process culminated in my career as a surrogate.

In addition to my story, I relate many of my clients' stories because I believe they have much to teach us about sexuality and the issues that can complicate it. Their experiences provide a rare window into what really drives and heals sexual problems.

If it isn't already evident, I suppose I should confess that I have a mission with this book. I hope that it will, even in some small way, encourage open and honest discussion about sexuality. I also hope that it will inspire readers to claim and honor their sexuality at every age. Everyone has a right to satisfying, loving sex, and, in my experience, that most often flows from strong communication, self-respect, and a willingness to explore. It is my goal to inspire the frank and fearless consideration that can lead to all three.

1.

heavy breathing: mark

....

Mark O'Brien opened his mouth slightly, making a little silent hiccup. I grabbed the tube that sprouted like a plastic tendril from the portable respirator his aide had clamped to the headboard. As I sat up to bring it to Mark's mouth, my breast grazed against his cheek and we both smiled. Mark squeezed his lips around the flat mouthpiece of the tube and the reassuring hiss of air filled his lungs. He closed his eyes. He luxuriated in oxygen, something most of us took for granted. The machine blinked and made loud ticking noises. He loosened his lips and opened his eyes. I gently removed the tube, leaving it on his pillow, just outside the crescent of sweat that rimmed his head. "How are you feeling?" I asked. "Good, Cheryl. It wasn't as scary as I thought, or it was, but I'm still glad I did it." Then he flashed his sweet, boyish smile.

It was 1986 and I had been a surrogate partner for thirteen years. I had worked with disabled clients before, but none as compromised as Mark. At thirty-six, Mark had lived most of his life in an iron lung after having contracted polio at age six. He could only breathe on his own for short periods of time and it was only with the help of the respirator that he could meet with me for a couple of hours in the spacious Berkeley cottage he had borrowed for our first session.

The iron lung was essentially a breathing machine. It looked like a wide pipe with levers and dials that encased Mark's whole body, leaving only his head exposed. It worked by creating a partial vacuum every few seconds that lifted his chest so his lungs could fill with oxygen. Because Mark slept in the iron lung, he didn't own a bed. Luckily, he had a supportive friend who was willing to share hers with us.

Except for the ability to wiggle a few fingers and toes and move his mouth and eyes, polio had left Mark paralyzed. It had also contorted his body so that his left hip twisted to the right, jamming his legs together in a way that almost made them look fused. His neck and head were frozen to the right, making him gaze permanently off to the side. He spent his entire life lying flat on his back, except for when he was propped up for an attendant to wash or dress him or a doctor to examine him.

Like all of my clients, Mark was referred to me by his therapist. Like most of them, he was anxious in the first session. "This is a big day for him," Vera, one of Mark's attendants, said when I arrived at the one-bedroom cottage that morning. The friend who owned the cottage was also disabled so the cottage was outfitted with a ramp at the front door and low kitchen cabinets and door handles.

Vera led me past the living room skirted with bookshelves that were low to the ground and down a hallway lined with black-and-white landscape photographs. She knocked on the bedroom door at the end of it. "Mark, Cheryl's here. We're going to come in," she called out before slowly opening the door. She motioned for me to go in first. Mark lay on a broad four-poster bed covered up to his chin with a blue afghan. Sondra, Mark's therapist, had told me that he was slight, only four-foot-seven and around seventy pounds and for a moment I was startled to realize how small that really was. The blanket that covered him was barely raised off the bed. "Hi Mark," I said, "it's so nice to meet you." "Nice to meet you, Cheryl," he said in his gurgly voice. His cornflower blue eyes stared downward.

"Just let me show you how to use the respirator and I'll leave you two alone," Vera said. She pointed out the small switch that I would need to flip on to start the flow of oxygen and then she put the breathing tube into Mark's mouth. "See?" I nodded. Mark took a few little gulps of air and released his lips. "He'll let you know when he's done." She took the tube out of Mark's mouth and said, "I'll see you guys a little later."

From the way he said my name, Che-ryl, I could tell that Mark and I had something in common. We were both transplanted New Englanders. I told him I was from Salem, just outside of Boston, and that I had been born into the big French Canadian community there. My maiden name was Theriault (pronounced "Terry-O"). " . . . Or 'There-ee-alt' if you were one of the Irish Catholic nuns at my elementary school."

"You're Catholic?" he asked.

"I was," I said, and smiled.

"I still am," he said. "I need to believe in God so that I have someone to yell at."

I laughed and Mark's eyes brightened.

I took off the jacket that I really didn't need on this warm mid-March day, dragged a chair from the corner of the room, and sat down by the side of the bed. "Let's talk a little about how we'll work together," I said, as if I entirely knew. Like therapists, surrogate partners have a protocol and a repertoire of exercises to help clients effect change in themselves and their lives. These obviously would have to be tailored to Mark's condition, and I wasn't entirely sure I knew what that meant. "We'll work at your pace. What I'd like to do today is learn more about you, and, if you are ready, start with a body awareness exercise," I said.

I asked Mark to tell me a little about his family and his childhood. He was born in the Dorchester section of Boston and had moved with his family to the Sacramento, California, area when he was sixteen.

He was the oldest of four children. He had some memories of his life before polio. He remembered waking up excited every day to run outside and play. He loved the outdoors and playing with the kids in the neighborhood.

When the disease struck in 1955, Mark was six and he became the focus of the family, especially for his mother. Her dedication to him was unwavering. She cared for him with patience and tenderness throughout his young life.

A few years after falling sick, Mark's sister, Karen, died of pneumonia and since that time an unearned guilt had shadowed him. He believed that his parents, particularly his mother, were so preoccupied with him that they didn't notice that Karen needed help until it was too late. Even though there was no reason to believe this was true, Mark still burned with guilt. He felt guilty about other things too.

Mark sometimes woke up with his crotch sticky with semen. He remembered a flicker of disgust cross his mother's face as she cleaned him one morning when he was around twelve. He could get aroused by having his left leg edged further over to his right so that his penis was sandwiched between his thighs, and a few times he had asked his attendants to position it this way. He discovered this accidentally when an aide had left him like this for a few moments while bathing him.

Even though Mark could hardly be called a traditional Catholic, he still felt shame about his sexuality, which he attributed to his religious upbringing. Like his guilt about his sister's death, it may have been irrational, but to him it seemed as real as the imposing iron lung in which he spent most of his days.

His parents never talked about sex and he received no education about it from the rafts of doctors and therapists who treated him throughout his life. Like many disabled people, Mark's sexuality went unacknowledged. Most people seemed to assume his disability canceled out his need for touch and intimacy.

Despite all of his physical challenges, Mark had earned a bachelor's degree in English from the University of California, Berkeley, and was a published poet and journalist. He tapped out his work using a mouth stick and a word processor. Mark had started on a master's program in journalism before the effects of post-polio syndrome, a condition that attacks the muscles and causes debilitating fatigue, forced him out of it. He lived near campus and traveled to and from school on a reclining wheelchair that looked like a motorized gurney. He lay flat on it or slightly propped up. His spine was too curved for him to sit up in a standard wheelchair.

Mark had felt alone and alienated for as long as he could remember. Most days he could imagine no end to the loneliness that stretched out before him like a boundless, desolate road. His sexual experience consisted of a few furtive touches from nurses and sudden arousal while his attendants bathed him. Embarrassment always followed. "Sometimes I let myself think that there is someone out there for me, but, really, I think it's hopeless. I feel like I'm outside a fancy restaurant, looking through the window and watching people feasting on all kinds of wonderful food that I'll never be able to taste," he said.

I had been a surrogate and a student of human sexuality long enough to know that attraction involves many factors and you need not have a pop culture–approved body to have a loving relationship and a sizzling sex life. I knew other disabled people who enjoyed both. Still, was he right about not being able to find a partner? I found myself thinking. Even though I had only just met Mark, I felt real affection for him. He was witty, smart, and brave, but could someone this profoundly physically impaired realistically expect to find a partner? Would I date him, or would I be too scared? By training and by temperament I'm inclined to be supportive and encouraging, to see possibilities and potential even in tough situations. I wanted to reassure Mark that there would be someone for him, but I also worried about creating false hope.

"Mark, I can't predict the future, but part of my job as a surrogate is to prepare you to have a loving, happy relationship if you meet the right woman," I said. "Let's talk more about what you want to get out of this process and let's learn more about what your body is capable of." I think I said this as much to be honest with Mark as to remind myself of what I could and could not do as a surrogate partner.

"Suppose you began a relationship with someone tomorrow who you thought was just perfect. What would you feel?"

"Well, probably a lot of things. Anxiety, excitement, relief."

"What would the anxiety be about?"

Mark paused and then asked me to bring the oxygen tube to him. I stood up, the redwood floor of the old cottage creaking as I took the few steps to the respirator. After a few seconds he slackened his lips and I took the breathing tube out of his mouth.

"That it would be obvious that . . . that I'm a virgin and she would want someone more experienced and capable."

"Okay, so it's important for you to get some experience. That's natural. Lots of people worry that they won't have enough practice to please a partner."

"I don't want to live my whole life without having sex."

"You don't have to. We can accomplish that together."

For someone like Mark to be told that what he wanted was achievable and that his fears were not so different from those that many of us confront was reassuring. Even clients who don't suffer from the kind of physical challenges Mark faced are often relieved to hear that they are not alone in their insecurities and worries. Mark was so accustomed to being an outsider, to being someone who needed special consideration and accommodation that hearing this probably felt akin to a compliment.

Mark and I had talked for close to an hour, and, if he was ready, it was time to begin the physical part of the session.

"How would you feel about doing some physical exploration now?"

"Okay, I mean, yeah, I'd like that."

It was time for us to get undressed and this would mean me taking off Mark's clothes and seeing his body for the first time. Suddenly, I was scared. He was so fragile. What if I hurt him? What if I couldn't maneuver around his body? Go slow, slow, slow, I told myself.

"Mark, if at any time I'm doing something that doesn't feel good,

let me know. This is important not just for our work together, but for
you to learn how to express likes and dislikes to a potential partner.
If something feels bad or uncomfortable, just tell me to stop, okay?"

"Okay," he said, with a slightly worried look on his face.

"Remember, this all happens at your pace, so if you want me to
slow down or stop at any time all you have to do is tell me."

I slowly lifted the blanket that covered him. His frail body was in
a red, long-sleeve, button-down shirt and a pair of black sweatpants.
Slow and gentle, slow and gentle, I said to myself, like a mantra. "Let's
start with your shirt." I undid the first button and then worked my
way down the column of buttons. When I was finished, I undid the
button at the wrist of his left sleeve. Then I folded his shirt over his
arm as much as I could. The collar rested off his shoulder. Because he
spent so little time outdoors, Mark's skin was pale. Against the red of
the shirt it looked salt-colored. I briskly rubbed my hands together to
warm them up and then slid one under his shirt. I carefully brought
Mark's delicate arm toward me while inching the sleeve off of his
shoulder. As I continued to peel it away, I moved his arm back down
toward the bed. The sleeve was almost completely off when Mark
screamed—loudly. Oh my God! Had I hurt him?

"What's going on?" I said in as calm a voice as I could muster.

"My nail, you caught my nail in the shirt," he said.

"Okay, okay . . . let me see." I freed his fingers from the shirt that
was now clustered around his hand.

Remember to ask Vera to trim his nails, I told myself.

"Mark, I need to know when something doesn't feel good, but
yelling isn't sexy. I know we need to be very careful with your body, so
don't ever not tell me if you're feeling uncomfortable or worried about
getting hurt, but try to do it in a calmer voice. Remember, part of what
we're doing here is modeling how you'll communicate with a partner,
and that could really scare someone and kill the mood." I had goose
bumps on my arm that I hoped Mark didn't notice. "Do you need
some oxygen before we go on?" To my surprise, he didn't. Once I had
freed his left side from his shirt, I went to work on the right.

Then it was time to take off his pants. Mark's left hip jutted up and over like a hood of bone and a sliver of his left butt cheek was exposed. At seventy pounds, he was light enough for me to slide the elastic waist of his pants and underwear down past his groin and knees while he stayed pressed flat against the bed. When I got to his feet, I gave the pants a little tug and they came completely off of him. Then I saw his fragile, exposed body in full.

"How are you doing, Mark? Are you warm enough?"

"Yeah," he said in a low voice.

It was my turn to undress. I took off my blouse and jeans, unhooked my bra, slid off my underwear and socks, and draped my clothes over the chair as Mark looked on.

"I've never been with a n-n-nude w-w-woman before."

Even though his body was skeletal, Mark had a chubby face and it turned pink.

"That's why I'm here," I reassured him.

I got into bed next to him.

"Most clients are really nervous at this stage," I said. "A big part of having satisfying sex is being able to relax, so I'm going to show you an exercise that will help with that."

The point where Mark and I were in our work together was were I would typically teach my clients how to do deep, diaphragmatic breathing in which you draw full, long breaths in, expanding your abdomen, and then immediately but slowly exhale as you deflate it, all the while trying to focus solely on your breathing. I also generally guide clients to do a full scan of their body, encouraging them to free any tension that they detect. Because Mark couldn't breathe fully, however, I asked him to concentrate on each breath he took, even if it was shallow. "Close your eyes and try to clear your mind of everything but your breathing," I said.

We lay next to each other for a few minutes with our eyes closed and our minds trained on our breath. I rolled over to my side and snuggled next to him, the heat of his body warming my breasts and thighs. At five-foot-eight, I felt nearly Amazonian next to Mark.

"Doing good," I said. I gently placed my arm over his waist, slightly tensing my muscles so that my full weight didn't rest on him.

In first sessions I typically do an exercise called Sensual Touch. I think of it as a close reading of a client's body. I explore him from his toes to his head with my hands and observe all the particularities of his physicality. I notice skin tone, temperature, freckles, scars, and the other attributes that make each body unique. Sensual Touch gives clients an opportunity to begin to learn about which areas of their body are the most responsive. Clients are often surprised to find that areas outside of the genitals can feel arousing or pleasurable to my touch. For example, more than one client has told me that the backs of his knees are a particularly sensitive area.

I explained Sensual Touch to Mark. Although he was paralyzed, he still had sensation all over his body, so he would feel my hands moving up and down. Typically, I explore both the back and front of a client's body, but with Mark I was limited to the front and the left side of his back because of the way he needed to stay positioned. I encouraged him to try to recognize four common reactions: feeling neutral, feeling nurtured, feeling sensual, and feeling sexual. "Sensual feels pleasurable, but not necessarily sexually arousing. Sexual is arousing. There are only two rules: Do your best to stay in your body and in the moment, and let me know if something doesn't feel good. When you realize that your attention has drifted, bring yourself back into your body, to where my hands are."

I ran my fingers through Mark's hair and told him how soft and wonderful it felt.

I slowly got up and walked to the end of the bed. I took his feet in my hands. They were narrow and slightly clammy, and his toenails were a bit too long. I made another mental note to ask Vera to trim his nails. I lightly kneaded the balls of his feet with my thumbs and he wiggled his toes.

"Does that tickle?"

"No, it feels good," Mark replied.

I worked my way over the tops of his feet to his ankles and up his shins, which had only a sprinkling of down-soft light brown hair. I slowly swept my hands over my thighs and inched my way up to his groin. Mark was already hard and his scrotum was bulging and had turned a deep brownish red. I gently took his penis in my hand and circled around it lightly with my fingertip. As I released it and started up his abdomen Mark let out a little yelp and came. He squeezed his eyes shut and said "damn it" under his breath. Then he said, "I'm sorry."

"Don't worry. It's okay," I said.

It was clear that Mark was going to need some help in prolonging ejaculation, and this gave me a perfect opportunity to explain the human sexual response cycle and the arousal scale.

"The human sexual response cycle has four stages. The first is Excitement, which begins with the first twinge of arousal. It's when physical signs like erection happen. Plateau comes after that. This is an exquisite stage that can be prolonged. You're fully aroused at this point. You may notice some pre-ejaculate and you'll typically see some muscle tension and your heart rate will pick up. The third stage is Orgasm; and the last is Resolution, when your body returns to its pre-arousal state." I explained to Mark that we would try to prolong the Plateau phase.

In order to keep himself in Plateau longer, Mark would also have to understand the arousal scale. "The arousal scale measures where you are in the Plateau stage. It goes from one to ten. One is the very beginning of arousal and ten is orgasm. It can be difficult at first to recognize the gradation, but with practice it gets easier, and it's a good tool for prolonging arousal," I said.

I grabbed a few tissues from my handbag and gently wiped away the semen from Mark's penis and surrounding area. It was time to finish Sensual Touch.

I traveled up Mark's abdomen to his chest and up his neck. I dragged my fingertips over his Adam's apple and the left side of his jawbone. I circled around his eye and then down his nose and chin. Carefully, I made my way to his feet again.

When I finished exploring the front of Mark's body, I walked to the top of the bed and started down the sliver of the left side of his back that was exposed. I traced my fingers over the shoulder blade and then down the arm. I returned to his back and lightly brought my hand down it and around his left buttock.

Then I returned to bed. "Can you tell me what parts of your body felt the most sensual?" I asked.

"It felt great when you touched my shins and my face, but to be honest, most of it felt sexual to me." I wasn't surprised to hear this. When people have been starved for touch and their sexuality hasn't been recognized, their bodies can become acutely sensitive and any touch anywhere can feel arousing. My sense was that as touch became less foreign to Mark his body would respond to it in more complex and nuanced ways.

Mark asked if he could kiss my breasts. I lay on my side and softly brought my left breast to his mouth.

"Now, the other side," I said in a tone of pretend seriousness.

I tipped my body over so that Mark could kiss my right breast.

Then he made the gulping motion that I'd come to realize meant he needed air. I hoisted myself up on my elbows and slid the breathing tube into his mouth. He drew a few breaths, smiling as he took in the air.

❧

Three weeks later at our next session, the first thing I noticed about Mark was that his hair hung a little longer. "I didn't get it cut because of what you said the last time," he said. I remembered that I had commented on how silky his hair felt. I ran my hand over his head and said, "It feels just as wonderful as it did then."

The bedroom window overlooked a bed of daffodils that spring had just started to pry open and I felt a bit sorry when I unrolled the shade and blocked them out.

Mark seemed calmer this time, and, frankly, I was too. The goals that we were striving for and the issues we would address were now much clearer to me than they had been in our first session. I would try to help Mark lose his virginity and also help prepare him for a happy sex life if he found a partner. I still wasn't convinced that a long-term relationship was in Mark's future, but I could help him feel more confident if it was.

We chatted a bit about our last session. Mark said it was a little like going to college in that he could think of a hundred reasons why he couldn't do it, but he did it anyway and he was happy he did. He also told me that he was at work on an autobiography and he planned to write about our time together. Then he announced that he wanted to try something new this session.

"I want to do something to pleasure you."

"Well, I won't argue with that."

It's not unusual for clients to want to give me pleasure. It's a natural impulse. Most people don't want to simply be passive recipients. They want to give as well as receive pleasure. As a general rule, unless it is something that doesn't feel good to me or is something I think would interfere with the goals of the work, I allow clients to touch me when they ask. If a client has difficulty communicating with a partner about what she likes, it can be a perfect opportunity to model a conversation about her preferences.

Even before I undressed Mark I could see that he was fully erect. When I slid off his pants they caught at his stiffened penis and I had to stretch out the elastic waistband to move them past his groin. I undressed myself, and just as I was about to climb into bed Mark cried out, "Oh God, oh God, oh God," and came.

Mark's face turned so red that it looked like poppies had exploded under his cheeks. "It's okay, Mark. Really." I lay down and wrapped my arms around him for a few minutes. I could feel the rapid thump-thump-thump of his heart. "Do you remember the breathing exercise we did the last time?" We closed our eyes for a few moments and concentrated on our breath. I felt his pulse slow a bit.

I ran my hand down Mark's arm.

"You said something about pleasuring me," I said.

Mark gave a little half-smile, seeming to overcome his embarrassment. "I like your nipples. Do you like to have them sucked?"

The truth was that I loved it, but for a second I flirted with claiming the opposite. What scared me was that Mark would stop breathing while he sucked my breast. The tabloid headline, "Suffocated by Breast," flitted through my mind. I looked over at the respirator and the breathing tube that lay inches from his lips. I could do this. I would do this. "I love it," I said. I straddled Mark's narrow frame and pressed the palms of my hands down on either side of his head. I would have to do a push-up-like motion to lower each of my breasts into his mouth. I placed all of my weight on my left hand and then lifted my right to make sure I could balance on one hand if I had to quickly grab the breathing tube.

"I could think of worse things to choke on," Mark said.

Slowly, I bent my arms and shifted my hip to the left so that I could lower my right nipple into his mouth. Mark tightened his moistened lips around it and pulled in.

"That feels really good."

After a few seconds I lifted my breast out of his mouth to ask if he needed air.

"No, I need nipple."

This time I lowered my left breast into his mouth and he took it in more intently than I had ever seen him draw in oxygen.

When I lifted my breast out of his mouth, Mark asked if I would scratch the area behind his testicles. I reached my hand down and told him to tell me exactly where he wanted me to touch. When I put my finger on his perineum, the strip between the scrotum and the anus, he said "there." I scratched lightly and Mark said "harder." I applied a little more pressure and he moaned with delight.

I buried my head in the crevice between Mark's left jaw and shoulder for a few seconds, and then he asked if we could have intercourse.

I asked him to check his breathing for a few moments. I reached for the condom in my purse and quickly put it on him. I straddled Mark and lowered my pelvis down to brush his penis against my mons. Before I could get him in me, Mark came again.

"It's okay, it's okay," I said preemptively.

Mark closed his eyes and squeezed his lips. His cheeks turned pink.

"It's okay," I repeated.

I stroked his hair and he opened his eyes and smiled.

Then his eyelids started to drop and he became dreamy, a look I would come to see always followed his orgasms.

I do my best to stay in the moment with my client, but lying next to Mark that day, I noticed myself worrying about our next session too much to be entirely present. That's because the third session is typically when I do the mirror exercise. It is one of the most telling exercises in surrogacy work and it involves the client standing before a full-length mirror describing how he feels about his body. As we lay quietly together, I started mulling over just how I would adapt this for Mark. I worried about how he would react. Was he ready to do this? I was just about to broach the topic when he asked if I had ever read Shakespeare's "Eighteenth Sonnet."

"Many years ago, in school."

"Well, I memorized it for you."

"Shall I compare thee to a summer's day?" he began.

"Some air," Mark said as he finished the first line. I brought the breathing tube to his mouth and he let the oxygen fill his lungs. He parted his lips and I took away the tube.

"Thou art more lovely and more temperate/Rough winds do shake the darling buds of May/And summer's lease hath all too short a date . . . "

Clients had expressed appreciation before, but never with a love poem that has endured centuries. I snuggled against him and I realized how much I hoped that Mark would find a partner and that one day he might lie next to her reciting this very poem.

Boundaries can get fuzzy in surrogacy work. Having sex, even in a therapeutic context, invariably creates attachment between people.

Early in my career I worried about how to maintain a professional degree of distance and still create the intimacy that is so vital to the surrogacy process. It can be a tricky balance, and I was concerned about clients bonding with me when one of our main goals is to help them build healthy relationships in the "real" world. Had we met in my early years as a surrogate, I think I would have been concerned that Mark was becoming unhealthily close to me. But thirteen years into my career I had seen enough to know that expressions of gratitude generally don't signal anything more than a client wanting to show sincere appreciation.

"So long as men can breathe or eyes can see/So long lives this and this gives life to thee," Mark finished.

"Mark, that was beautiful. I want you to know how much I've liked getting to know you and how happy I am that we're working together."

I ran my finger over the ridge of his hip and down his leg. I felt myself becoming more aroused than I had been in all of our time together. It is not uncommon for me to get turned on when working with a client. This doesn't mean, though, that I necessarily progress to intercourse or that I act on my arousal in other ways. Surrogacy is client-centric and the physical interaction is geared toward achieving his goals.

Alongside my arousal, I felt a pang of sadness. Mark was such a sensitive soul, and he could make such a fine lover for someone. I hated to think that he wouldn't have that opportunity. I wanted to resume the touching and tenderness, but I knew I had to discuss the mirror exercise with him.

Given how polio had twisted his body, I wasn't sure he had ever seen his adult genitals. Even though I was anxious about how he might respond, I still believed that it was important for him to see his body in full.

"I'd like to discuss our next session," I said. "I'd like to bring a mirror so you can really see your whole body. How does that sound?"

Mark hesitated. I was getting used to the clues his body transmitted, and I could feel his skin heating up and warming mine. Understandably, this was sensitive ground for him.

"I don't know. I'm curious, but I'm afraid of what I might see."

"What scares you about seeing your body?"

"I've never actually seen my dick," he said. "What if it's deformed?"

"You have a perfectly normal penis, Mark. You'll see."

What worried me wasn't Mark's reaction to his penis, but to the rest of his body. Would he be shocked to see himself naked for the first time as an adult, in the aftermath of polio?

I took his face in my hands and kissed him on the forehead. Mark parted his lips and his Adam's apple bobbed up and down. He needed air. I flipped the oxygen switch on the respirator and brought the hose to his mouth. He drew deep breaths from the cloudy, ribbed breathing tube.

"Thank you, Cheryl," he said when I took it away from him.

As I drove home that night I began to feel a lot less anxious about our next session. Like many of the disabled people I had worked with, Mark was resilient and courageous. He could handle seeing his whole body. Maybe he would even be happier than he thought with it. Besides our Catholic upbringing and New England roots, Mark and I had something else in common: I hadn't seen my genitals until I was an adult either.

℅

As the 1970s dawned, I was living in the San Francisco Bay Area, and, along with many others, I was actively questioning just about everything I had been taught. I enrolled in a masturbation workshop taught by the wonderful Betty Ann Dodson, Ph.D., (or Dr. BAD, as we lovingly sometimes called her), the author of the groundbreaking *Liberating Masturbation: A Meditation on Self Love* (later retitled *Sex for One*) and *Orgasms for Two*.

The day started with a trip to the grocery store. Betty guided the class of about twenty women to the produce aisle and had each of us select a zucchini. After that we headed to a classroom that was lined with overstuffed pillows. Betty had brought a hand mirror and we each took turns propping ourselves against a few of the pillows and looking closely at our vulvas. Betty also invited the students to look at each other's vulvas. She had a flashlight to help us better see one another, and when she asked if anyone wanted to volunteer to hold it, I raised my hand. I didn't think I would ever get an opportunity to see the genitals of so many different women, so I jumped at this chance. If a student was willing to show her vulva, I pointed the flashlight at it so the class could get a clear view. It turned out that no one was unwilling, and all twenty women shared their vulvas with the class. Many of the women were surprised to realize how beautiful female genitalia is, and to see the similarities and differences among us. With much laughter, we each noted which size zucchini we had picked and what it suggested about our size preference. Then there was a discussion about how we masturbated. Some used a vibrator or a dildo, and others simply used their hands. Most cared less about the size of what went into her vagina, and more about how she was stimulated and touched. I still remember the excitement that charged the room. To see so many women discovering the beauty of their genitals is something I'll never forget.

When I do the mirror exercise, I sometimes see that my male clients have a similar response to Betty's students. It's one of the reasons I think the exercise is so important, and eye-opening. For some it's the first time that they have thoughtfully looked at their own bodies. I hoped that Mark's reaction would be at least something like mine was on that day with Betty.

Because we couldn't use the cottage where we had met for our first two sessions, Mark borrowed another friend's home for the third.

Dixie, another of Mark's attendants, let me in and pointed to the back of the apartment. She noticed the mirror sticking out of my tote bag. She paused for a moment as though she were going to ask me about it, but then she smiled shyly and said, "Just through the kitchen and to the right." It was a small apartment with peeling paint on most of the walls. The kitchen counters had been covered with the same green linoleum that was on the floor. As I made my way back to the room where Mark was waiting, my shoes stuck a little and it felt like I had to peel them off the ground with each step.

I knocked on the heavy oak door of the bedroom. "Mark, it's me, Cheryl." Then I slowly opened it and walked in. This time, the mattress was on the floor. There was a desk scattered with papers in one corner of the room. Mark's feet stuck out of the blue afghan that covered him. They were clad in socks that were as white as eggshells. His feet never touch the floor, I thought, and felt a prickle of guilt. A shaft of light streamed in from the big window that faced the University of California campus and a blizzard of dust danced in it. Mark smiled. "Great to see you again, Cheryl," and, then, before I could respond he added, "You brought the mirror."

I sat down on the mattress and kissed Mark on the lips. When I lifted my head back up, I swept my long, brown hair across his chest.

"I did. A little later we'll do the exercise we discussed last time, okay?"

I asked Mark how he had been in the three weeks since our last session. His writing career was keeping him busy and he had just landed an assignment from a local newspaper to write an article on disability laws. He had been looking forward to today. He was starting to think that he could have and enjoy sex like a "normal" person. What's more, he had given me sexual pleasure. For someone like Mark, whose sexuality was treated as an inconvenience at best, this was a real confidence booster. Like most of us, Mark wanted to know that he could delight someone in bed.

I undressed him and then myself. As always, Mark lay on the far left side of the bed. Because his head was permanently turned to the right, this ensured that he could see me when I lay next to him. I sat down on the right edge of the mattress and hoisted my legs onto it. Then I rolled over on my side and cuddled up next to him. His penis was already erect. I kissed him on the top of his head. "You're already able to stay in the Plateau stage longer. That's progress." I caressed his face and chest. I kissed him on the lips and scratched his perineum and scrotum. I noticed that his scrotum was lifting, a sign that he would soon orgasm. I stopped touching and asked him to check in on the arousal scale. "Can you estimate where you are, from one to ten?" I asked. He said he thought he was at about seven. Then I asked him to practice the breathing technique I had taught him. I put my hand on his thigh and moved it to his penis. A squeal of delight blossomed into a howl and he came.

"I didn't want to do that yet," Mark said, frustrated.

"It's okay. Remember last time? You can probably have another orgasm."

"I wanted to have intercourse today."

"Let's see if we can."

I ran my hands slowly down Mark's body and back up again. I took his face in my hands and kissed his nose and then his mouth. Then I positioned myself so that my legs were on either side of Mark, giving him easy access to my breasts. He licked them, tensing his tongue and circling around the nipples. I took his hand in mine, and folded his fingers so that they made a fist. I then guided his hand to my genitals and gently rubbed his knuckles against my clitoris. "I really like to be touched like that," I said. I reminded him that some women want a different pressure, so it's important to start off lightly and then ask if they want more.

Mark grew hard for the second time, and I quickly covered his penis with a condom. "Let's just put the tip into me and see what happens." I took his penis in my hand, and moved it around my vulva. Then I inserted the head into me. I asked him to pay attention to his level of arousal. I didn't move at first, and then I pressed down on his shaft. About a minute passed before Mark orgasmed.

"Did you come?" Mark asked. When I said I didn't he was disappointed, but I reassured him that we could try again.

"How did that feel?"

"Okay, I guess. It was so quick."

"Yes, but you were inside me. This is a big step, Mark."

He smiled and then closed his eyes, drifting in his gauzy, post-orgasm reverie for a little while. When he surfaced again, I asked if he was ready to take a look at himself in the mirror. It was time for Mark to see his genitals for the first time in his adult life.

I propped up the mirror horizontally on the far edge of bed and stood behind it, holding on to the middle of its three-foot frame with my fingertips. I tilted it back slightly so that Mark could get a full view. He was silent for a few seconds. He scanned up and down his body.

"What are you thinking?" I asked.

"Not bad. Better than I had imagined."

I was so relieved.

In surrogacy work the victories are small and incremental. It may not sound like much, but Mark had made definite strides. He was able to sustain an erection a little longer and he had grown more comfortable with himself and his body. Even though he couldn't use his hands without my help, he learned to work with his mouth and tongue to pleasure me. That started in the first session when he took my breasts into his mouth, and by the last he had progressed even further. With luck, this would come in handy with a future partner.

Three weeks later on a hot July day, Mark and I met for our last session. Dixie yelled "come in" when I knocked on the door and she led me into yet another bedroom in the apartment that had a pile of clothes in one corner and a desk with an imitation Tiffany lamp that gave off an amber light in the other.

"You brought the mirror again," Mark said when I entered the last of the borrowed bedrooms where I would see him.

"I'd like you to see your penis hard."

I undressed Mark and myself. Mark's penis was again already erect, so I took the mirror to the side of the bed to give him a view of himself aroused.

After he motioned to me that he was finished looking, I climbed into bed next to him.

"What do you think, seeing your penis this time?" I asked.

"I think it's alright, really alright," Mark said and smiled.

I held him for a few minutes and then he asked if he could taste me. I knelt over him and slowly lowered my vulva to his mouth. He kissed it softly and then pushed his tongue in. He swirled it around my inner labia and pushed it into my vagina. He moved it in and out rapidly and then sucked with his lips. He kissed my clitoris. It felt wonderful. After a few seconds I pulled back and brought the breathing tube to his mouth. I was aroused. When Mark signaled that he was done, I moved the breathing tube back to the respirator. I snuggled up next to him and circled my leg over his hips, feeling his penis poking into my thigh.

I put a condom on Mark and then brushed my finger around the head of his penis and squeezed the shaft lightly. Then I straddled his body so that his penis was inside of me. I began languorously moving up and down. My vagina started to flutter. I had also reached a high level of arousal. I slowed down to prolong the Plateau stage for both Mark and me. I breathed in and out and then remained still, asking him where he was on the arousal scale. "About eight," Mark said. I kept still for another minute and then lifted myself up so that the shaft of his penis was partially outside of my vagina. Then I eased down and pulled up again. Mark orgasmed. He had stayed aroused and inside of me longer than he had in any of our past sessions. Even after he came Mark remained hard enough for me to move up and down again and achieve full orgasm myself.

He asked almost immediately if I came. When I told him I had, he beamed.

"Do you need more oxygen?" I asked.

"No. I actually don't," he said. "If only this counted as respiratory therapy, maybe I could get SSI to pay for it." We both laughed.

Polio had caused Mark's chest to be misshaped. It tented up a little and was hairless. I leaned forward and tenderly kissed it. Mark gulped and I grabbed the breathing tube. "No," he sputtered. I realized that he was crying. "No one's ever kissed my chest," he said. Then my eyes filled with tears. "It's about time they did."

⌒

Mark stayed in touch with me on and off for years after our final meeting, and I was delighted when, in 1994, eight years after our first session, he called to let me know he had met someone. Susan first became aware of Mark by reading some of his poetry online. She was so moved by his words that she emailed him. An online relationship was born and soon it evolved into a real-life one. Mark was tickled that his fear of never finding anyone had been proven wrong, and he was thrilled to have entered the relationship with some experience behind him. "Thanks to you I didn't have to say I was a virgin," he said.

2.

the sin under the covers

....

My work has given me enough stories to fill this and any number of other books. Some, like Mark, center on people with extraordinary lives and challenges. But most are of those who grapple with more straightforward concerns, like erectile dysfunction or premature ejaculation. When I chip away the particularities and personal eccentricities, I almost always find that much of what they struggle with on the deepest levels are issues few of us would find alien. Loneliness, anxiety, fear, guilt, or shame about sexual feelings, low self-esteem, poor body image, and body ignorance are just a few in the constellation of all-too-common issues that I see every day.

My career as a surrogate now spans close to four decades and includes hundreds of clients. I consider myself blessed to have found this profession when I did and to be able to know that what I do changes people's lives for the better. It has been a long and rich career. When people ask where and when I started, I answer 1973, in the San

Francisco Bay Area, but that's only partly true. Really, it started at least two decades before and three thousand miles east of California.

The city of Salem, Massachusetts, lies sixteen miles north of Boston on the coast. Salem Neck and Winter Island extend out from it like two fingers stretching into Salem Sound. By the time I was born in 1944, Salem had been cleaved into ethnic neighborhoods. The Polish, Italian, Irish, and French Canadian communities were largely composed of the descendants of immigrants who arrived in the nineteenth century to work in the city's textile mills.

My family members on both sides made their way from France to Canada and then down to Massachusetts, bringing their French language and customs with them. Luckily, they also brought their recipes. My great-grandmother on my father's side was a wonderful cook. When we went to her house, mouth-watering aromas of French food greeted us as soon as we crossed her door—including her specialties: cipate, a casserole layered with vegetables, meat, and pastry dough; creton, a pork pâté; and bouef bourguignon.

Salem is a place with deep ties to and constant reminders of its past, especially the Salem Witch Trials. The Witch House, home of Judge Jonathan Corwin, one of the judges appointed to hear some of the first charges of witchcraft in the late seventeenth century, still looms eerily at the corner of North and Essex Streets. Gallows Hill, where around twenty innocent women were hanged after being caught in the crosshairs of hysteria and religious fundamentalism, isn't far from my childhood home. These days the city capitalizes on its history for tourism dollars and witchcraft kitsch abounds, but when I was growing up witches were no Halloween marketing ploy. To my child mind, they were very real. They served as warnings to stay on the right side of God—or at least the Church.

I was the first child born to Virginia and Robert Theriault. Almost two years later, my brother David came along; eight years after that my brother Peter arrived. With his job at the New England Telephone and Telegraph Company, my father earned enough money for my mother to be a full-time homemaker. He started out as a salesman selling advertising for the yellow pages and later became a manger. Unlike most of his counterparts in management, my father didn't have a college degree. He did, however, have a gift for art and for gab. Both of which helped him in his selling days. As he talked up particular ad opportunities for clients he would draw out what they would look like, bringing them to life on the sketch pad he took on all of his sales calls.

For the most part, my family was made up of hardworking, decent people. Many of them were inclined toward generosity and, for the most part, they were a lively and fun bunch who delighted in big family dinners, music, dancing, storytelling, and laughter.

Growing up, the person I was closest to was Nanna Fournier, my grandmother on my father's side. She was funny, intelligent, and kind, and she was crazy about me. One of my earliest memories is bolting out of my stroller so I could run into her open arms. She also had a sharp fashion sense, and as I got older I was the only girl I knew whose grandmother gave reliable advice for looking hip.

For all of their merits, my family members were also people of their times. They were steeped in a rigid Catholicism and a pre-women's movement mentality about the proper role of women. A woman's job was to look pretty, win a stalwart husband, and then be a doting wife and mother and make a comfortable home.

My mother took this job seriously. Impeccably neat, slim, well-coiffed, and—frankly—obsessed with appearance, she never cut anything less than an attractive figure. She also kept an immaculate home and was often frustrated by what she considered to be a lack of appreciation on everyone's part. As good as she was at it, I don't think my mother ever enjoyed being a homemaker. She was often angry, and, in retrospect it's easy to see why. The Valedictorian of her high school class, this bright and capable woman must have secretly yearned for more and felt unfulfilled with the endless cycle of cooking and cleaning and childcare that made up her days. At the time, though, all I knew was that no matter how perfect she or the house looked, my mother always seemed dissatisfied. "Didn't anyone notice . . . "

she would say in exasperation after polishing the floor or washing the drapes or performing some other thankless domestic task.

When it came to sex, the religious, cultural, and social forces of the time converged to create a code of silence that could only be breached to issue harsh judgments and condemnations, usually aimed at women who had in some way transgressed. On one occasion my mother made it a point to note a woman in town, a former classmate of hers, who was "loose." From the tone her voice I could tell that being loose was something very bad. Before I was even sure what it meant, I knew that I never wanted to find myself in this category of women.

My mother couldn't even say the word "vagina," much less talk about anything that might go into it. To her, it was a "hoosie," and that was only when she absolutely had to refer to it. As for sex education, or at least what passed for it at the time, they left that to the nuns and teachers at St. Mary's Immaculate Conception Elementary School, which I entered when I was five.

Ꙅ

In second grade, my class started receiving training to make our first Holy Communion and preparing to make our first confession. The Baltimore Catechism served as our manual to all that was good and holy. Sometimes I was afraid to even look at this hallowed book, with its diffuse picture of Jesus and his sad, benevolent eyes staring out at the fallen world from the cover.

We learned the difference between mortal and venial sins and I had my first introduction to the sins of impurity. We were taught that touching "down there" was one of the gravest of mortal sins. It was a particular affront to God and anyone who did it was corrupting body and soul and risking eternal damnation. This conjured up all sorts of terrible hypotheticals. What if you touched down there and then died before you could confess? Of course, you would be hell-bound. I vowed never to touch myself in an impure way. I would keep my soul pure, even as I flailed in the temporal world.

Soon after starting school it became clear that something was different about how I learned. Much later, when I was an adult with two children, I would be diagnosed with dyslexia, but at the time my difficulty in learning how to read, write, and do math was taken as defiance, laziness, or just plain stupidity.

My classmates learned how to put sounds together and decode words and then sentences with what seemed like barely any effort. I was stumped by one-syllable words like "dog" and "cat."

My mother enlisted herself in the effort to help me learn how to read. She promptly went out and purchased a series of "Dick and Jane" books and we had regular tutoring sessions after school. Each day we sat at the kitchen table and I would try to read the adventures of Dick and Jane and their dog Spot. My mother was no more enlightened about dyslexia than my teachers and less patient than some of them. I don't know if she thought it would prompt me to learn faster, or if she was frustrated, or if she thought I was willfully misunderstanding basic concepts, but she resorted to physical punishment.

The afternoons with her devolved into a predictable and frightening cycle: She would tell me to read a word, I would read it incorrectly. "Sound it out," she would demand, and when I still misread it she would grab my arm and squeeze it so hard that I sometimes cried out in pain. Once, she became so enraged after I misread "can" three times that she lifted me off my chair by my arm and then slammed me back into it. I started having so much anxiety that the words on the page blurred when I tried to read them, which made my performance and my mother's anger worse.

What I couldn't understand and what I would resent for years was that my mother was an otherwise compassionate woman. We had a neighbor Greta who was mentally handicapped. I had seen my mother be so gentle and kind with her. I had seen her insist that Greta be treated with dignity and respect. And it wasn't just with Greta that my mother showed tenderness. She was a good neighbor who readily helped anyone who needed a hand. Why couldn't she show any sensitivity to me? Did she know that there was something bad about me? I figured I must have been fundamentally unlovable and in need of drastic improvement. Trouble was, no matter how hard I tried, I couldn't seem to better myself.

I was probably in third grade when I concluded that something about myself had to be kept secret. I had come to believe that I was what was then called "retarded." I just didn't show it like Greta did. I had to keep it quiet or I would never be allowed in the same classroom as my friends—that is, if any of them still wanted to be my friend after they found out. I would become a social outcast and an embarrassment to my family. Nanna Fournier was the only one who would probably stand by me, but I wouldn't tell her. She might still love me, but imagine her disappointment if she found out. Certainly no one would want to ever marry me if this got around. On one hand, I thought I was lucky not to be obviously retarded. On the other, I suspected I might be better off if I were. Then, at least, people would lower their expectations and I wouldn't disappoint them.

At the end of each school year, I dreaded the terrible news that I would have to repeat a grade. To my relief, it never came. I managed to squeak by from year to year. Maybe it was to compensate for my academic deficiencies, but I soon became a real cutup, and at times a devilish one. I could chat with anyone and loved to talk. I was, by nature, an optimist and even a leader, at least on the playground. I learned that I was funny and had a knack for socializing and story-telling. I could reenact movie scenes, reeling off the dialogue in the voice of Natalie Wood or Tony Curtis or any of the other popular movie stars of the time. I could make my classmates laugh and they liked me for it.

‌ℬ

By the time I reached junior high, I couldn't always hide my poor performance in school, and my friends started to help me keep pace with the rest of my class. Often before heading off to school we met at Martha's Sweet Shop around the corner from St. Mary's. Martha's had a soda fountain and played the latest and hippest rock and roll. Elvis, Buddy Holly, Bill Haley and the Comets, the Big Bopper—my friends and I swooned over them while we enjoyed Lime Rickeys and English muffins smothered in butter and jam. My compatriot Lisa and I would sit next to each other on the stools that swiveled all the way around and she would carefully go over my homework, replacing my mistakes with the right answers.

Unfortunately for me, our morning cheat sessions didn't last beyond the first few months of the eighth grade. One chilly morning as "Chantilly Lace" blared from the jukebox and Lisa and I huddled over my math homework, I spun around and saw two dark figures approaching the door, their habits swirling around them like smoke. As they got closer there was no mistaking them: Sister Agnes Gene-vieve, my eighth-grade teacher, and Sister Alice, the Mother Superior. Somehow they had found out about the pre-class homework swap-ping at Martha's, and they put an end to it that day. Even though I worried about how I would now eke out passing grades, I was partly relieved that the sisters had intervened. Cheating was, after all, a sin—one that I could now ill afford since I had begun committing the queen mother of sins: masturbation.

Since the concept of self-esteem had a long way to go before it would become part of the popular culture and something that good teachers would be careful not to undermine, most nights I was racked with anxiety about the humiliation the next day might bring, and unable to sleep. Unfortunately, the antidote was a mortal sin.

Starting when I was around ten, I masturbated and brought myself to orgasm nearly every night. It was the only thing that helped me relax and fall off. If my nights began with anxiety, my days began with guilt. I became convinced that every earache, every toothache, every injury was God punishing me. Later, I had painful periods that often kept me in bed. These, too, I thought were God's judgment. I couldn't escape his gaze or his wrath. Sometimes I imagined my guardian angel looking away in disgust as I touched myself and rocked back and forth in my bed.

I had displeased God and my Guardian Angel. Not to mention, my mother. One evening she caught me masturbating and bellowed, "Get your hands out from under the blanket now!" as she stood in my bedroom doorway.

The priests to whom I confessed were equally appalled. Every Saturday afternoon as I reeled off the "Our Fathers" and "Hail Marys" that were supposed to absolve me of the sin I committed under the covers, I pledged, again, to resist temptation. My confessors let me know that I was guilty of a particularly vile sin and that I was doing nothing less than letting down Jesus Christ himself with my unwillingness to resist it. They were disgusted and disappointed with me. Soon, they would have even more reason to feel this way.

3.

irreconcilable differences: brian

....

Father Dennis had a baritone voice that made him sound like he spoke for God himself. In the confessional his full-throated announcement of penance carried with it as much condemnation as salvation and I dreaded it so much that my voice shook as I listed my sins, which invariably included masturbation. But that was a long time ago. It was part of a childhood policed by a God who was as vindictive as he was omniscient. A God, who, by 1976, I no longer believed in. Still, it was Father Dennis's bottomless voice that I flashed on as I listened to Brian, a client who came to me in the fall.

I was three years into my career as a surrogate partner at that time and one of around one hundred in the profession. Today there are few trained surrogates in the United States. The International Professional Surrogates Association (IPSA) puts the number at fifty. Even in the late 1970s, when the numbers were at an all-time high, I would estimate that there were no more than two hundred of us, most living and practicing on the coasts.

Brian met me in the one-bedroom apartment I had converted into an office. I used the living room as a consultation room and the bedroom for the physical part of my work with clients. When I decorated the apartment I did my best to make it a place that clients would feel comfortable and at ease in. I had overstuffed chairs in the living room, and the walls were painted a soft peach. Fresh cut flowers often adorned the end tables and I usually made snacks available. The last thing I wanted was for a client to feel like he was in an austere, clinical environment.

At thirty-two, Brian suffered from difficulty achieving and maintaining an erection. His penis would only partially stiffen for a few short minutes before turning flaccid again. He had struggled with this since his marriage broke up two years ago, and it was easy to see why. Cecile, Brian's now ex-wife, was a devout Catholic and she divorced him because she had caught him masturbating in their bedroom one afternoon. I found it interesting that she was willing to overlook the Catholic ban on divorce, but not its prohibition on masturbation. I never met Cecile, but I wondered about the agony she must have felt at having to weigh the sin of divorce against the sin of masturbation and make a choice that would leave her religious conviction, not to mention her immortal soul, intact. In this difficult reconciliation, it was clear which evil was judged the lesser.

Brian was short and stocky. He owned an auto mechanics shop that he had worked hard to build into a thriving business. He sat in the easy chair across from me and bounced his leg up and down nervously. He recounted the day Cecile stumbled upon him in the act. "She only wanted it once a week, so I used to do it a lot. I usually did it in the shower or at the shop after everyone went home," he said. "But that day, I was in the bedroom. It was a Saturday and she was out in the garden, so I thought she'd be outside for a while and that I was safe."

He had almost climaxed when Cecile opened the door and screamed, "What are you doing?" Brain scrambled to get on his pants, covering his penis with his hand. "It was like I was ashamed not just because of what I was doing, but of being naked, of my body."

Cecile made Brian sleep on the couch that night. The next morning she told him that what he was doing was a sin and it was perverted. He was a married man. He should have outgrown his need to masturbate. If he loved her, he wouldn't do this.

Not only had Cecile imbibed the Catholic dogma about masturbation, she also harbored one of the more persistent myths about it. She believed that once you got married, you "matured" sexually and that meant leaving masturbation behind and transferring your sexual energy to your spouse. Sure, it was 1976, the sexual revolution still had some steam left, and it was the progressive Bay Area, but old myths die hard.

A few awkward weeks passed before Cecile announced she wanted a divorce. Brian pleaded with her not to leave. He promised he would never touch himself again. He offered to go to counseling. All of this left Cecile apparently unmoved, and before the end of the year the divorce was finalized.

As we made our way through our first session, Brian talked a lot about Cecile. I had a strong sense of what she thought, but what did Brian think? Did he see himself as guilty? "I don't know. I don't think she would have left if I wasn't doing something terrible," he said. "I destroyed my marriage over . . . that." He ran his hand through his honey-colored hair. "I know that I haven't been able to have a real erection since she caught me. It's been two years now and I keep hoping it's going to change."

"It's sounds like you are punishing yourself," I said.

"Probably," he said.

"Brian, it's unfortunate Cecile is so misinformed, and maybe one day she'll get better information, but you did nothing wrong. Masturbation is natural and healthy."

"Even if you're married?"

"Married, single, divorced, engaged, cohabitating. Yes, there's nothing wrong with masturbation."

I think Brian knew this on some level, but hearing it from me reinforced it. Surrogacy work often begins by assuring people that sexual impulses are no cause for shame. Brian's thoughts were ambiguous, at best, about what he had done. He may not have believed self-pleasuring was a marriage-killing sin, but he was far from comfortable with it. I asked him to tell me his views on masturbation and what he had been taught about it.

"I was raised Catholic, so I was told it's a sin. I guess I never wanted to believe that. No one ever discussed it in my family or anywhere else. I don't know. A lot of my friends think that a real man doesn't need to do it because he has a woman."

I assured Brian that those ideas were myths, too, and I asked him what happened when he started to become aroused and touched himself.

"I start to fantasize, but then I catch myself and shut it down. Then I get anxious about whether or not I'll ever be able to have another hard-on. The irony is that I haven't been able to masturbate since Cecile left me."

He added that since the divorce, the few times he had been with a partner had ended in embarrassment and apologies for not being able to "perform." This humiliation and the fear that he would never have another relationship spurred him to see the therapist who eventually referred him to me.

"I have a homework exercise for you," I said. "I want you to give yourself permission to fantasize. Try to initiate fantasies throughout the next couple of weeks and try to give yourself the okay to continue with them. Remember, they are just fantasies, so they can be anything you want—they can be immoral, illegal, or fattening—anything."

Like many clients, Brian was in a bind. I could sense that he was curious and wanted to separate sexual fact from fiction. On the other hand, he was so guilt-ridden and afraid of sexuality that even learning more about it felt wrong. Clients frequently arrive with plenty of opinions, feelings, and attitudes about sexuality. The problem is that too often they are forged by cultural fallacies, media-generated stereotypes, and plain old lies. I continue to be amazed at how solid education delivered without judgment can eradicate much of the guilt and shame that turns life in the bedroom into a struggle instead of a pleasure.

I asked Brian if he was ready to try some physical exercises. When he said he was we headed to the bedroom and got undressed. I peeled away the quilt on the bed and invited him to lie down. Then I got into bed next to him.

As always, I started by teaching Brian some relaxation exercises. I asked him to take long, slow, deep breaths that inflated his stomach and then full exhalations that returned it to its normal shape. I had him close his eyes and I guided him verbally through a mental scan of his body from his head to his toes. "Continue breathing, and when you find a tense spot in your body breathe into it and then breathe the tension out with the next exhalation," I said. When we finished the scan, I guided Brian in another five deep breaths. "Try to release any remaining tension." I asked Brian how he was feeling, and he said he felt more relaxed than when he had arrived.

It was time to move on to Spoon Breathing. This exercise deepens intimacy and brings me into contact with a client. I asked Brian to turn to his left side so that his back was facing me. Then I turned over so that I was snuggled up against him, spooning. I draped my arm over his waist and bent my knees into the backs of his. "Just breathe naturally," I said softly. "Take nice, easy, normal breaths." I paid close attention to the rhythm of Brian's breathing and synchronized my own with his. Soon we were breathing in and out together and a physical and emotional synergy started to build. I asked Brian how he felt and if he was ready to go on to Sensual Touch. When he said he was I asked him to roll over into the middle of the bed onto his abdomen and spread his legs into a V shape. I knelt down on the floor below the end of the bed. I asked him to take a deep breath, and when he exhaled I started exploring his feet and ankles. He had low arches and calluses around the outer edge of his big toes.

I moved to the bed and knelt between his legs. The hair on his legs was almost white, lighter than the hair on his head. At first, he was so tense that the muscles in his thighs and back felt like rope. As I slid the palms of my hands over them, I could feel some of the tension subside. I passed my hands over his butt and up his back. He had cinnamon-colored freckles across his broad shoulders. I went across each shoulder and then down his arms to his hands. The tautness in his muscles unraveled a bit.

I moved back up his arms to his shoulders and neck and then I reached the crown of his head. I rubbed the exposed side of his face, tracing my hand along his cheek and jaw, circled his ear, and then headed gingerly down his body again with broad-handed strokes. I traveled down until I reached the balls of his feet. I gently squeezed them and asked Brian to take a deep breath. As he exhaled, I let go. In a voice that was just above a whisper, I asked him to roll over onto his back when he was ready.

I gradually worked my way over the front of Brian's feet, over his legs and to his groin. When I touched the shaft of his penis, it stiffened and the muscles throughout his body tensed. I asked him to take a deep breath as I let my fingers ascend to his pubic mound, abdomen, and then his chest. I ran my fingers over his shoulders, arms, hands, and then back up to his neck and face. I circled his eye orbits. I touched his forehead, ears, lips, and jaw. Then I started down his body for the final time.

Throughout Sensual Touch, Brian's penis was never totally flaccid. His erection grew and diminished and then grew again. I often see this in clients, and at this stage it is not appropriate to have intercourse with them. A big misconception about this work is that the surrogate and client have sex immediately and in every session. One of the major goals of surrogacy, especially in the early stages, is to help the client become more aware of and in tune with his entire body. For him to have an erection and then lose, regain, and lose it again is helpful because it gives both him and me information about what arouses him and what doesn't. Intercourse comes later, after we have experienced a number of other exercises and gradually increased the level of intimacy between us. The intention here is for him to learn more about what turns him on and to understand that his erection will return when he is in an erotic mindset and not worrying.

Two weeks later, Brian sat across from me in my office. His shoulders were high and he fidgeted with his hands. He picked almost obsessively at a bowl of nuts on the coffee table.

"How are you?" I asked.

"I don't know. The homework—I couldn't do it. I just can't clear my mind enough."

"That's okay. Remember, we're just at the very beginning of our work together. Try to be patient and compassionate with yourself."

"I'm not sure I can change. Just when I start to get hard I panic and it goes away."

"There's every reason to believe you can change, but it won't happen overnight. You'll build the skills that will help, but it takes time. Remember, try your best to be patient with yourself."

We talked a little more. Brian recalled other fallacies he had grown up with. Too much masturbation would make you blind. It was a sign of mental illness. It could become a dangerous obsession.

"All untrue, Brian. Masturbation is natural, and it's good for you—in many ways. It strengthens the prostate, relieves stress, and helps you to better understand your own sexuality. I have another exercise I'd like to show you today, one that'll help you become more settled in your body."

Kegel exercises build the pelvic floor muscles and increase sensation in the genitals. When done regularly, they can make arousal and orgasm more acute. Kegels are probably more often taught to women, but they are also useful for men. They are used in surrogacy to help clients develop "sensate focus," the ability to be intensely aware of and attuned to physical sensations, especially the muscle tensing that comes with arousal. I thought if I could help Brian's mind become more in tune with his body it might change the messages it sent.

We left the consultation room and headed to the bedroom. We slipped off our clothes and lay beside each other on the bed. I explained Kegel exercises to Brian. "They help tone the puboccygeus, or PC muscle. The best way to identify this muscle is to try to cut off the flow of urine the next time you are in the bathroom. When you do this, you're using your PC muscle. Try it the next time you're peeing. When you ejaculate, the PC muscle kicks in involuntarily."

Then I walked him through the exercise.

"Imagine that you are sucking deeply on a drinking straw. Take a long breath in through your mouth and count to three, and, as you do this, tighten your PC muscle. Imagine that you have to pee, but aren't near a bathroom. Hold it for a count of three seconds and then let your muscles relax. Then take short, quick breaths, so that you inhale when you tighten and exhale when you release. Alternate between the two methods. Repeat the deep breathing twenty times, and then do the quick breathing twenty times."

We ran through a few cycles of the exercise together and I suggested he start with sixty repetitions a day in increments of twenty and work his way up to one hundred.

We did Sensual Touch again, and this time Brian seemed more at ease. As I worked my way up and down the back and front of his body, I noticed less tightness than I had in our earlier sessions and at times it seemed as though Brian was close to asleep.

When we were finished, I asked him for feedback. He told me that his shoulders and feet felt sensual, and his lower back and genital area felt sexual. He felt nurtured when I caressed his arms and the backs of his legs, and he felt neutral everywhere else.

As is typical in the second session, after I was finished exploring Brian and had heard his feedback, he explored me.

I rolled over onto my abdomen and Brian knelt on the floor. He took my toes and feet gently in his hand. I could tell almost instantly that Brian had a wonderfully sensual touch. As he made his way up my body, it also became evident that he had paid close attention to how I had touched him. He used similar, full-handed, slow strokes.

Brian glided his strong hands up my ankles and the backs of my legs. He lightly circled my hips and butt and then traveled to my lower back. He applied a little more pressure and the tightness in my muscles gave way to his touch. With his hands spread out, he went up my back and to my shoulders, down my arms and to my hands. Then he went back up my shoulders to my neck. He used his fingertips to softly trace around my forehead, down my nose, and around my cheeks and lips.

He went down my body a second time. When he reached my feet, I turned over at his request. As Brian slowly inched up my body, I became more relaxed and arousal started to build. He softly raked his fingers over my pubic mound. Brian sensed my muscles tensing and gently pressed his palms into my abdomen as I took deep breaths. His hands continued up, and when he got to my breasts he took his index finger and circled around my areolas. When he reached my face, he slowed his touch down even more. He lightly dragged his fingers over my lips. Then he smoothed along each side of my nose and over my cheekbones. He made it to the crown of my head and then started back down my body, revisiting all the areas he had touched previously. Then, without any prompting, Brian asked me if I was ready to give him feedback.

I told Brian that I felt nurtured almost the whole time he had touched me. It felt sexual when he touched my inner thighs, breasts, face, neck, buttocks, nipples, and inner arms. It felt both sensual and nurturing when he touched the rest of me. I didn't feel neutral at any time. Brian then lay down alongside me, our hips and shoulders touching. I felt the heat of Brian's body. We closed our eyes and started deep breathing. A few cycles into it, I opened my eyes and noticed that Brian's penis had become harder.

I sensed the trust between Brian and me deepening. Brian had now touched me and he knew that I enjoyed it. This often helps a client feel like they are on more of an equal footing with me. We continued to breathe deeply for a few minutes, and when I opened my eyes to talk to him, Brian's penis had relaxed.

"Brian, are you ready to get up?"

"Yes," he said in a sleepy voice.

I got out of bed and asked him for a hug. As we let go, I thanked him for the experience. Then we got dressed and walked up the corridor and back to the consultation room. I reminded him to practice the Kegel exercises he had learned and we made an appointment to see each other again two weeks later.

By the time we finished our third session, Brian had made steady progress. He was now regularly practicing Kegels and the breathing and relaxation exercises I had taught him. His fear and guilt around masturbation had diminished and the length of time he could maintain an erection jumped to five or six minutes, almost twice what it had been. He reported that he was able to melt into his fantasies a little more and that he noticed subtle changes in how he thought. For example, he still might find himself saying "stop" when he started to become aroused, but he no longer felt that he had to act on that command. Practicing the relaxation techniques helped him to recognize and relieve the anxiety that short-circuited his erections. This was a lot to accomplish in three sessions, but it was in our fourth when Brian really turned a corner. That's when we did the Sexological.

Brian arrived at our fourth session with a smile on his face. He had made more progress than he had thought possible. He had even considered asking a woman out on a date. After we talked for a little while, I ushered Brian into the bedroom.

"The Sexological is an exercise that focuses on the genitals," I explained. "We'll explore each other in depth and give feedback as we go along. There are two ways that this exercise can be helpful. First, it gives you an opportunity to really discover where in your genital area you're most sensitive and receptive. Second, it helps to take communication to a more intimate level. You'll tell me how you feel all throughout the exercise and then when it's my turn I'll do the same. The goal is to eventually be able to have this kind of conversation with a partner."

Brian tensed up a bit.

"The Sexological is deliberately clinical. The only thing we're trying to do here is pay close and careful attention to how we feel. I'll ask you about this as we go along. There are no right or wrong feelings. It's just thoughtful, slow exploration. Try to stay in the moment and in your body. Use your senses. Really take in what you're seeing, smelling, tasting, hearing, and feeling. Many people don't get erections during the Sexological. Some do. Either is natural."

I turned on the lamp on the nightstand. Then I went to the closet and pulled out six pillows, four to prop against the headboard, which Brian would lean back on, and two for me to support myself in the middle of the bed. I pulled out a hand mirror, tissues, and lubricant from the nightstand.

I took off my trousers and button-down shirt and then I swept my hair back into a barrette so it wouldn't get in the way. Brian got undressed and I took him by the hand and led him to the bed. I asked him to sit up against the pillows at the headboard and keep his knees bent. I adjusted the pillows to give my lower back support while sitting in the middle of the bed between his legs. I stretched my legs into a wide V and then asked Brian to do the same, and to put his legs over mine. When he did this our legs made a diamond shape.

Brian's legs were bulky with muscle and the hair on them slightly tickled my knees. He had broad shoulders and short fingers and a long scar down his forearm. His abdomen was divided by a line of hair that thinned out and disappeared before reaching his chest. I took his hands in mine. "Deep breaths," I said. Together we inhaled and exhaled a few times until I flexed my fingers and we uncoupled our hands.

Brian's penis was of average length. His pubic mound was covered with a wide triangle of blonde hair. His large scrotum spilled out beneath it. "Remember, Brian, as we go through this exercise, you have permission to have or not have a hard-on," I said. "However you react is okay."

I bent at my waist, took Brian's penis in my left hand, and lengthened it out with my right. I folded it up gently against his pubic mound.

I slowly glided my fingertip along the glands that make up the head of his penis. I went up the right side, around the top where the urinary opening is, and then down the left side.

I felt the muscles in his legs tense. I suggested he let them relax. Every time I felt an area of his body tense, I placed my hand on that area and asked him to release the tightness.

"Tell me how that feels. Does one side feel more sensitive than the other?" I asked.

His neck and face turned rosy and I could see the muscles in his abdomen becoming taut.

"I think the right side, but I'm not sure," Brian answered. I went around the head again and asked him if he could feel a difference now, reminding him if that if he didn't it was perfectly fine.

"I'm still not sure."

"Okay, let's keep exploring."

I touched the frenulum, the triangular area between the head and shaft of the penis, then I ran my finger between the two glands. I asked Brian how that felt.

"Good. Really good."

I went around the coronal ridge, which is located at the very edge of the head of the penis and asked him how that felt compared with the other areas I had touched.

"Not as sensitive as the one before."

"The frenulum?"

"Yeah, the frenulum is more sensitive."

Brian's penis was starting to stiffen. I held it with my left hand and made three strokes up and down on the right, middle, and left just below the head. I did the same at the middle of his penis and just before the base. I asked Brian for feedback at each section and he told me that being touched on the right side just below the head of his penis felt best.

I did the same movement on the right, middle, and left of the scrotum and asked Brian to tell me how each area felt. I ran my finger along his perineum. Then I traced the Raphe line, the seam that forms when the fetus differentiates into a male, and runs from just below the head of the penis to the scrotum. Like many men who are circumcised, Brian's Raphe line was crooked and veered right. Brian told me that his perineum was more sensitive on his right than anywhere on his Raphe line.

Brian's breathing started to quicken and I asked him to close his eyes.

I smoothed a little lubricant on my hands. I closed my fingers loosely around the base of his penis and twisted my wrist as I moved my hand upward toward the head. I did this spiraling motion first with my right hand and then with my left. I asked him if one felt better than the other. He said that he felt more excited when I used my left.

Brian was fully erect and his scrotum tightened. I asked him to take a few deep breaths and then I led him on a scan of his body so he could identify and loosen tight muscles. "It's natural to tense up with arousal, especially in the abdomen, butt, and thighs, but letting go will help you prolong this feeling you have now," I said.

I snatched one of the tissues that lay next to my thigh and wiped away the lube.

"Now I'm going to use my mouth," I said.

I bent further at my waist and took his penis into my mouth. I arched my knees slightly to make it easier to bend. Because Brian's legs were over mine, they raised a little as I did this and he tensed up.

"Relax your legs onto mine. Let me do the work here," I said.

He released his muscles and his legs rested loosely on mine.

I swirled my tongue around the shaft and the head. I could feel it against the roof of my mouth. I withdrew so that my lips pouted around the head of his penis. Then I released my lips.

"How does that feel?"

"Good," Brian took a deep breath. "Great, actually."

"Did you prefer the oral or hand stimulation?"

"Oral."

I sat up so that my back made a straight line. This is the point in the exercise in which I stop exploring the client and reflect on what we have discovered. Together, Brian and I gained a lot of knowledge about where his body was most reactive and sensitive to stimulation.

"I just learned a lot about where you like to be touched. Your frenulum, your perineum, the right side of your penis—these are all very sensitive areas for you. You also really responded to oral stimulation and liked it when I swirled my left hand down your penis. That's a lot to work with."

I asked Brian if he was comfortable and if he needed to use the bathroom or wanted a break. When he said he was okay, I asked if he was ready to explore me, and he nodded.

I slipped my legs out from underneath Brian's. A layer of sweat had collected between us and my legs glided out easily. I placed them on top of his, so that our legs continued to make a V shape, but mine were on top now.

I handed Brian the mirror and asked him to turn it to the magnifying side.

With my fingers I spread my large labia so that the rest of my vulva came fully into view.

"So, if you take the mirror and position it right about here you'll be able to get a good look," I said, pointing to a spot on the bed. "I'll take you on a tour of my vulva."

I put a little lube on my finger.

Starting at the top of my vulva, I pointed out my clitoral hood, my clitoris, and my small labia. Then I noted my urethral opening. Brian asked if it was sensitive. I answered that I don't enjoy having it stimulated, but that's not true of all women, so always ask a partner. I also reminded him to wash his hands before touching his partner's genitals so he didn't introduce bacteria and to be sure that his fingernails were cut short with no rough or sharp edges.

I pointed to just below my urethral opening and said that my G-spot is on the other side of this. "It's on the periurethral sponge, just about an inch inside on the roof of my vagina."

I showed him the vestibule, the area just before the vaginal opening and noted my hymenal remnants, which look like four raggedy skin tags located on the top and bottom of the vestibule. Then I inserted my finger into the opening.

I took my finger out and moved it along my perineum.

Brian was breathing heavily and I saw that his scrotum had moved up closer to his body. His penis leaked pre-come. I asked him how he felt. "Good, but a little scared," he said. When I asked why, he told me that he was afraid he was going to come too soon because he hadn't been with a woman for so long. It had been two years since he had last had intercourse and his attempts had ended in frustration. I reminded him that he had stayed fully hard for about fifteen minutes now, longer than he had in a while. Then we took a few deep inhalations. I asked him to release any tension in his abdomen, butt, and thighs on the exhale. His erection relaxed, and we moved on. I invited him to put a little lube on his fingers and to start exploring me.

I lifted my clitoral hood and asked him to touch my clitoris. "Mmmm . . . that feels really nice. Some women find direct touch too intense, but I like it. It's a good idea to start on the side of the clitoral hood and ask your partner if she likes to have her clitoris touched. She may not in the beginning, but that may change as she gets more aroused. Start with a light touch and then ask your partner to tell you how much pressure she likes. It's best to explore with lubrication, either natural or something bought."

I was starting to become aroused. I felt my butt and abdomen tighten and a flush of heat spread through my body. I took some deep breaths and released my muscles.

Brian moved his finger around the curve of my small labia. "That feels really nice, especially on the left side."

I asked Brian to insert his finger into me up until the first knuckle and to curl it up toward the roof of my vagina. "You're on my G-spot now. Mine is not as sensitive as my clitoris, but it still feels good to have it stimulated."

Brian explored me with his finger a little deeper, and I started to lubricate more. He moved his finger in and out slowly. "I'm noticing that I feel more on the right than on the left," I said. He eased his finger in deeper, until he reached my cervix. He asked what it was, and I told him. Then he asked if I liked having my cervix touched. I told him I didn't, but some women do, so always ask a partner how it feels to her. Brian eased his finger out. I took it, led it along my perineum, and told him how sensitive it is.

Then Brian closed his hand around the shaft of his penis and moved it quickly up and down. When he thought he was going to come, he stopped and did some deep breathing. He smoothed on some lubricant and then wrapped his hand around his penis again. He moved up and down more slowly for a few minutes and then picked up the pace. He cried "oh, oh, oh" and came. He leaned his head back against the pillows, his arms flopping out to the side.

"Brian, how do you feel?"

"Good."

He dropped his head to his right shoulder. He closed his eyes and his breathing became slow and even. I thought he was sleeping, until he said, "And not guilty."

I told him what tremendous progress this was and added that he now had a valuable skill at his disposal. "You are in complete control. If you want to prolong arousal and pleasure more before climax you can. It's up to you how long you want arousal to last."

Our fourth session was a turning point for Brian. It was the first time he had been able to masturbate himself to orgasm in over two years, and it was the only time he had done it with someone else present.

Like talk therapy, progress in surrogacy work is rarely linear. Often, we take two steps forward and one back. As a surrogate, I'm concerned that we move toward healing, and I expect to double back at times. This was the case with Brian. We began our fifth session with him telling me how he had once again begun to have difficulty maintaining an erection. "Frustrated, incredibly frustrated," he said when I asked him how he felt. I reminded him that overall he had made tremendous strides and assured him that setbacks are not uncommon.

"Try to be patient and compassionate with yourself. You're doing great. One setback doesn't negate all of the work you've done," I said.

In our remaining three sessions we did a number of other exercises. Brian pulled out of his slump and continued to improve. When he returned for his seventh appointment, he told me that he had been able to bring himself to orgasm several times.

At our last session he celebrated a month of guilt-free, satisfying masturbation and he told me about a wonderful woman he was seeing that Saturday night.

"I wasn't afraid to ask her out," Brian said.

"Fantastic! That's really great, Brian."

It is immeasurably rewarding to see a client become more confident and better able to connect with others in what I always hope will be a satisfying and loving way.

"Brian, I want you to know that if you ever have any questions or need some encouragement you're always free to call me."

Brian and I hugged.

"You're wonderful. Don't forget it," I said as he walked to the door.

Whenever I see a client overcome the kind of issue that Brian struggled with, I make it a point to note how far he has come and how much he has changed. For many years before I became a surrogate, I had to remind myself of the same.

4.

sex maniac

....

In my freshman year at Salem High School I came down with
the kind of flu that I thought for sure was a preview of my afterlife if
I didn't curb my nightly sinning. My throat was so sore and inflamed
that I could barely swallow. Both of my ears were plugged up and I
was chilled even beneath two quilts. When I coughed it felt like steel
wool was scraping out the lining of my throat. Getting out of bed
to go to the bathroom exhausted me. No way could I drag myself
to school. As a result I missed the first week of October, and when I
returned I had a pile of catch-up work to do.

On my first day back, I went up to a second-story science classroom to retake a lab. As I approached the door, a few lanky members
of the basketball team stood chatting in the hall. At fourteen, I was
self-conscious and shy. I would have never dared to talk to them. I
might have been a teenage raconteur with my girlfriends, but around
boys I became timid.

My outgoing personality may have masked it, but I harbored deep insecurities about my appearance. I didn't think I was pretty enough and I had plenty of complaints about my body, starting with breasts that I thought were too floppy. I wanted the ones that stuck out like rosebuds. When I compared myself to some of the prettier girls in school or the movie stars of the time, I came out painfully short. Around these high school jocks I instantly felt hyperconscious of my physical flaws.

One of the boys milling around the hall was a good-looking guy with short blond hair and blue-grey eyes. I walked past them and knocked on the door to the classroom, but no one answered. I waited a few seconds and knocked again. Nothing. Just then the cute guy walked over and knocked on the wall and, almost instantly, the teacher came to the door and let me in. "See?" he said, and flashed a bright smile. "Thanks," I said, wondering who the hunk with the magic knock was.

In those days dances were a popular social event. In the last week of October I attended the Freshman Frolic, which was held every fall in the gym at Salem High School. When I walked in Ritchie Valens's "Come on, Let's Go" was on the jukebox and a group of my friends were standing on the rim of the dance floor, sipping Cokes, laughing, and bopping to the music. Becky had on a teal strapless taffeta dress with a wide skirt and white high heels. Marcie wore an emerald green pencil skirt and a white collared shirt with a sweetheart neckline. I wore a red dress with a fitted bodice and a pleated skirt. In retrospect I think I probably looked pretty good, but at the time all I could feel was self-conscious about not being pretty enough, not sophisticated enough—not anything enough, except maybe for fat. I was definitely fat enough. Never mind that I was a normal weight; like many young women, I still considered myself too fat. I chatted for a few minutes and then I saw him. Actually, I think I saw her first. Judy Tolton walked by hand in hand with the guy from the hallway outside of science class. She had a chain around her neck with a ring dangling from it. "Hi Judy, hi Bill," Becky said when she saw them. So, now I knew his name. Of course, I also knew that he was going steady with the snootiest girl in town, and I guess I could see why. Judy Tolton, who had been in Miss Duffy's Dancing School with me for years but barely spoke a word to me, was gorgeous. She had lustrous beige-blonde hair that hung down to the middle of her back and pouty lips. She also had a slim waist and long legs. But what a snob! My heart sank. I slunk away to get a Coke. Since seeing Bill that day outside of my science classroom I had lost myself in fantasies that we would become a couple and that he would fall madly, hopelessly in love with me. It made me feel giddy with excitement. Now I just felt like a fool. I was only thankful that I had kept my longings secret. He was Judy Tolton's boyfriend. Judy Tolton, the girl everyone wanted to look like.

A few weeks later, when I had pretty much dismissed my fantasies of being Bill's dream girl, my friend Angela told me about Teen Town. Teen Town sprouted up every Saturday night at the Salem YMCA. You could dance, play pool or ping-pong, or just hang out. "It's so much fun. You've got to go," Angela said. When Saturday night finally arrived I put on a jersey dress, a bolero jacket, and pair of dressy suede flats. My stomach fluttered with nerves. The kids who went to Teen Town came from both the public and Catholic high schools and from all grades. At the time, mingling with seventeen-year-old seniors seemed pretty special. After all, they were within inches of adulthood and I was just out of grammar school. I checked myself for probably the tenth time in the mirror, got into my dad's car, and within a few minutes we were at Teen Town.

I scanned the room for my friends, and when I didn't see them I bought a Coke and sat down at one of the empty tables. Did anyone even notice me? What if none of my friends showed and I spent the night alone sipping Cokes. I was imagining just what a pathetic sight I would be when I heard someone say, "Wanna dance?" I looked up and there was Bill. I felt my stomach tighten. I took a deep breath, tried to settle down, and said "sure." We headed to the dance floor and Bill gently took my hand in his. It was then that he noticed I was

shaking and asked if I wanted to wear his jacket. I almost said yes so
he would believe that I was shivering from cold, instead of trembling
with nerves. He asked me my name and then asked how old I was.
I wished he hadn't because I wanted him to think that I was older
than I was. I confessed to being fourteen and asked him how old he
was. "Seventeen," he said. We started dancing and I felt myself loosening up a bit. Finally, I felt composed enough to ask him about Judy.
"Aren't you and Judy going steady? Why isn't she here?"

"Oh, we broke up."

Suddenly I felt like my whole body was smiling. "Oh . . . really,"
I said, trying to play it cool. Bill and I danced all of the slow dances
together that evening. When it was over he asked if he could drive me
home, but my father had already made arrangements to pick me up.
"Well, let me meet him" was his response. Whoa! This guy was really
confident. He was confident and sweet, a great combination. I introduced Bill to my father, and, to my delight, my dad said Bill could
drive me home from Teen Town the following week.

I couldn't wait to see Bill again. As I got to know him, I realized
how truly nice he was and how much he had going for him. He was
a star athlete. He played varsity basketball and baseball, and he was a
good swimmer. And was he cute! I couldn't believe my luck.

Looking back I realize that it wasn't exactly luck that drew Bill to
me. I'm fairly certain that Bill fell for me because of my personality.
After all, I was no Judy Tolton. If I could have remade myself then
it would have been in the sultry image of Kim Novak or Marilyn
Monroe or other popular actresses of the time. I thought of myself as
cute, but nothing special. I was vivacious and had energy to burn. I
am an extrovert by nature and I thrive on social interactions. In those
years, I was everyone's friend. My vibrant, outgoing personality was
my best feature, and I used it to the fullest extent I could. Other kids
wanted to be around me, and I often found myself at the hub of my
social scene. My energy was magnetic, and when they were around
me they had fun whether we were going to the movies, ice skating, or
just hanging out.

Bill and I soon spent every moment we could together. We not only had electric physical chemistry, but also a real friendship. I learned a lot about myself and what I liked with him. We spent hours in his car on Kernwood Road in the neighboring town of Beverly, where everyone went to park. It was wooded and just off the town's golf course. At the time there was a rumor going around that a rogue cop was pulling girls out of cars and raping them, but Bill made me feel safe. "I would never let that happen to you," he assured me.

It wasn't just the specter of a criminal cop that frightened me. My Catholic training told me that what I was doing was a mortal sin. I had taken the next logical and sinful step after masturbation. Once again, I was torn in two. Experimenting with Bill felt so good. He was almost as new to sexual play as I was and we fumbled around together, trying different things and having fun. We kissed passionately, exploring with our tongues. I had heard of French kissing before and now I was doing it. At the same time, I felt crushing guilt and shame. I wondered, again, why something that felt so good had to be so evil. Now, my Saturday confessions included two hell-worthy sins.

On one of our regular weekend night dates I wore a button-down sweater, and Bill and I created a little game. He opened the top button. There were, I think, around eight in all. We decided that I would wear something similar on each of our next eight Saturday night dates and each time we met he would undo one additional button.

I started to become concerned around that time by how much I really liked sexual arousal. I knew other girls were curious. My friends and I passed around books like *Tropic of Cancer* and *Lady Chatterley's Lover*, and we talked about sex, but it was always in an oblique way. We never discussed what we liked or what felt good or what we wanted to try. I assumed that my friends kept their hands above the covers at night and didn't feel the kind of excitement I did. No doubt, they wanted to know about sex, but I wanted to know about it and experience it. I worried that I was the only girl who really liked sexual feelings. What did this mean about me? If girls who did it before marriage were whores, what were girls who did it and liked it?

I didn't know the word for those girls, and I worried that I was the sole member of my gender who craved sex. For young women of this era, sex was currency and virginity was a bargaining chip. Your sex appeal wasn't about how much pleasure you could get, it was about what kind of man you could land. It was to be parlayed into a stable, monogamous future life. Virginity was not to be squandered on plea-sure. I couldn't stop exploring with my boyfriend, though. I started experimenting with touching Bill's penis. At first I just ran my fingers over the bulge in his trousers. Then I put my hand down his pants and held it. I didn't know what, exactly, you were supposed to do with these things, but I was learning.

Finally, the Saturday night came when it was time to undo the last button. We sat in Bill's car on Kernwood Road kissing and caressing each other. Then Bill ran his eyes up and down the stack of buttons on my shirt. We climbed over the white vinyl seats of his Studebaker. He undid the first seven buttons of my blouse. It was early spring and suddenly it struck me that we had gone from winter to spring in the course of eight buttons. We looked at each other and laughed. He undid the last button and I sat there in my bra, which he quickly unhooked.

Luckily, Bill couldn't fully see my body. The only light that filtered in came from the moon and the weak streetlight a couple of yards away from us. Also, I was lying back, which made me look slimmer than when I stood. Yet, there were also fleeting moments when Bill made me feel so beautiful that my insecurities melted away, and I was fully in the delightful moment.

Bill kissed my breasts and pulled gently at my nipples. I was already wet when he took off his pants.

I discovered with Bill that night that I loved finger fucking. I also learned that when I got really excited I got wet, wetter than I had ever gotten when I masturbated. Sometimes I worried I'd peed after a make-out session with Bill. Remember, this was the late fifties, when sex education for most girls consisted of "If you do it before you're married you're a slut." For Catholic girls like me it was "If you do it before you're married you're a slut and you'll fry in hell unless you confess."

He slowly slid his finger inside of me and my vagina started to pulse. Then he gently glided his finger out and slid his penis in. I panicked. Would I get pregnant? He must have seen the fear in me because he whispered, "I promise I'll pull out." I was so anxious that all I could think was that I wanted this to be over. I loved the foreplay, but penis-in-vagina sex had consequences so dire that I couldn't possibly relax enough to enjoy it. He thrust in and out of me and I held my breath. Finally, he pulled out and came on my mons. Oh, no! Did sperm have some kind of homing device that propelled it into the vagina? I tilted my pelvis up just to be on the safe side.

ꝏ

Bill and I started going "all the way" almost every time we could be alone. I wasn't happy about this. I was still terrified of becoming pregnant. I didn't know how to talk about this with Bill, or even if I had any right to turn back. I had already gone all the way with him. Some unspoken rule dictated that I couldn't hold out now. Bill knew as much about sex as I did. He was convinced that if we had intercourse during my period I couldn't get pregnant, so he came inside of me on those occasions. We were incredibly lucky. As much as I adored Bill, I also started to resent him. He wanted to have intercourse every time we saw each other, while I preferred the risk-free thrill of foreplay. Then I could relax and enjoy the electrifying sensation of arousal and usually I could have an orgasm by being stimulated by only his finger. But for Bill, sexual play had to culminate with his penis inside my vagina or he was unsatisfied. Since I had no vocabulary for expressing my sexual preferences and no belief that I had a right to, I quietly went along and did my best to keep my resentment under wraps.

Around this time, I started having a problem with my skirts: The zippers kept breaking. One Saturday as I sat in the living room reading a magazine, my mother came into the room clutching one of my skirts. "I don't understand how this keeps happening," she said, showing me the ripped zipper. "I told you," I said, "I broke it pulling it too hard in the bathroom." My dad, who was fiddling with the radio in the corner of the room, shot me a look that made it plain he didn't buy it. My zippers got torn in Bill's cramped, steamed-up Studebaker, not in a rush to pee. Dad didn't know this exactly, but he knew my excuse was fishy.

My father barely ever said a word to me about sex, but he still let me know his attitude about me having it. I remember one instance when I was sitting on the front porch with my parents, and my mother was recounting some shocking news she had heard earlier that day. Her friend Jackie's sixteen-year-old daughter was pregnant. When I heard this a chill ran down my spine. That could be me, and if it was I'd have to kill myself, I thought. Just then, as if he knew what I was thinking, my father looked squarely at me and said, "If you ever get pregnant, don't come home."

Often after sex Bill and I talked about what we hoped for in life. Bill always came back to one thing. He wanted to marry me soon. We would get an apartment and have a child together. He would go to night school and then we would buy a house with a yard big enough for a garden. Since we weren't using birth control, pregnancy was a constant fear for me. For Bill, it was simply an eventuality. If I got pregnant we'd get married immediately. We would tell my beloved grandmother and she would help us. If I didn't get pregnant we would get married the minute I turned eighteen. He explained that he wanted to be settled down with a wife and child by the time he was twenty-one.

Even though I was crazy about Bill, I didn't understand what the rush was. I was fifteen, still a child myself. I wanted to experience more of everything. I knew I didn't want to be married so young. I wanted to explore life, and—yes—have other lovers. If I married and had a child now I would choke any possibility of any of that happening. Yet, when Bill talked about marriage and children he seemed so sweet and sincere that I couldn't bring myself to tell him what I really thought.

I continued to go to confession every Saturday, usually with some of my friends. Now not only was I confessing to sex with myself, but with Bill, and I was judged not just for one odious sin, but two. The evidence that I was a very bad girl was mounting. I was breaking sacred law by myself and with someone else. I knew it was wrong, but I couldn't stop. It could only mean that I was inherently evil and weak. What's more, I had begun having thoughts that no decent person would entertain. I was secretly questioning much of what I had been taught about God. Why, I wondered, would God give us sexuality and then condemn us for acting on it? Why did only marriage sanctify sex? More broadly, I wondered how a book that was written by mere mortals could reveal the mind of God. Did this mean I was further incriminating myself in the eyes of the Almighty, or did it mean I was starting to think for myself? Was it the final step toward eternal damnation or the first stirrings of liberation? And what would liberation mean? Would it mean letting all this dogma go? If so, what would take its place? There was a war raging inside me, and it may sound melodramatic, but I really believed that if I chose the wrong side there would, literally, be hell to pay.

In the fall of 1959, Bill enrolled in a local college. We continued to see each other after school and on the weekends. I had worried that going to college would change how Bill saw me. He would be around older girls who were living more adult lives and would probably make me look like a kid, which, of course, I was. My fears turned out to be unwarranted. Bill seemed even more enthusiastic about us getting married and having a child after he started college. He would talk dreamily about what it would be like when we were married. I still couldn't see what his rush was. This didn't so much become a wedge between us, but more of a painful signal that we were headed in two different directions and neither one of us could change course. I tried to ignore it. I told myself that he would change. He would realize we were both too young to get married, much less have a child. He would let it go. Yet Bill continued to talk about it in the same loving, genuine way he always had.

I had to gather a lot of courage to finally tell him that I could not do what he wanted. One Saturday as we lay on the grass at Forest River Park, I looked him the eyes and said, "Bill, I just turned fifteen. I'm not even out of high school yet. I'm not ready to be a mother. I want to know more about life and to live more. I need other experiences—and so do you. If you can handle that and wait for me then maybe when we're older we'll get married. I don't expect you not to date. I'm sorry, but that's how I feel." I realized that I had just broken up with him, and so did he.

To my shock, a few days later Bill told me that he had left college and volunteered for the Marines. He would ship out to Paris Island for basic training within a week. I was flabbergasted. Why was he in such a rush? I was worried about him too. Bill was strong, but Marine Corps basic training was brutal. When I asked him why he did it, he just said, "I need to get my head straight." In the Marines? I thought.

When it came time for Bill to leave for basic training, I drove out to the recruiting station in Peabody with him and his parents. I felt awful. If something happened to him, it would be my fault. Then I would truly be a terrible person. We said a tearful goodbye and on the way back to Salem I was riddled with confusion. Had I made a mistake? Would I ever again find someone so nice who would love me as much as he did? Only a year ago I couldn't have imagined all of this happening. Life was unfolding fast.

It wasn't long before I met a boy who feared getting a girl pregnant about as much as I feared becoming pregnant. It happened, again, at Teen Town. John Leshky was known as a "good catch." He was a top athlete. A football quarterback, basketball star, and a respected track runner, John was also handsome and popular. He was tall and had intense hazel eyes. Emboldened by my experience in the dating world, I asked him to dance one night at Teen Town and we quickly became a couple. Being his girlfriend gave me a certain prestige among the other kids at school, and I liked it. Sometimes when the other girls looked at us I sensed a mixture of awe and envy that boosted my fragile teenage ego. As the girlfriend of one of the most revered boys in the social hierarchy of high school, I gained new respect among my peers.

John was a highly recruited athlete with scholarship offers from some of the top American universities. Everyone—including John—agreed that he was something special and a bright future lay ahead of him. The last thing he wanted was to get a girl pregnant and wind up a working stiff saddled with a wife and kids. Unlike Bill, he had no misty visions of a big house and a loving wife and child eagerly awaiting him at home. Perfect, I thought. No more panicking. No more resentment about doing something that I thought was way too risky just to please my boyfriend.

John was about as far from Bill in his temperament as anyone could get. Bill was sweet, charming, loving, and considerate. John was brash and arrogant. He could be fun, but he could also be cruel, especially if you weren't one of the kids who made up the galaxy of cool that swirled around him. He was also unlike Bill in that he wasn't much for rangy, thoughtful conversations. Our communication was generally superficial and unsatisfying. He wasn't my friend, much less my soul mate, which was what I yearned for. Still, there was a lot of physical chemistry and, best of all, I now had the most foolproof birth control on the planet—no intercourse.

This was around the time that I discovered the beatnik scene and started going to the Woodbury Tavern and the King's Rook, two local cafés where the coffee and the poetry flowed. Becky, Marcie, some other friends, and I started hanging out there our sophomore year. We would don all-black outfits, line our eyes with black pencil, and head out to one of the cafés to spend the night listening to poetry that was sometimes impenetrable, sometimes inspiring, and drink Italian sodas that came in exotic flavors like raspberry and tamarindo. It all made us feel supremely cool.

Sometimes I brought a notebook with me and tried to write my own poetry. It was pretty bad, but probably not worse than some of what I heard from the stage. Once, when I was at the Woodbury Tavern, I scribbled my name in my notebook and then wrote "Leshky" after it. "Cheryl Leshky," I said softly to myself. I didn't like the way it sounded. No, John wasn't my soul mate, or future husband. He was just someone who I could have a lot of great, worry-free sex with—or so I thought.

As with Bill, John and I spent a lot of time on Kernwood Road steaming up the windows of his car. The rumors of the rapist cop had dissipated. I still felt plenty of guilt and fear about what I might face in the afterlife, but I was at least certain I wouldn't get pregnant.

One night, John had barely put the car in park before we started kissing and grabbing each other. Along with being a great kisser, John also had a wonderful touch. Most of the time I got aroused the instant he laid a hand on me. John quickly slipped off my skirt and underwear and started masturbating me. Slow at first, then fast, then slow again. It was a rhythm that moment-by-moment brought me closer to climax. My self-consciousness fell away, and I disappeared into it. Slow, fast, slow. Then I had a mind-blowing orgasm, the first one I'd had with John. I moaned with delight. At that moment I loved him. Maybe he was my soul mate, maybe we connected physically in a way that was impossible otherwise. Would you know your soul mate by the strength of your orgasm? I couldn't keep it to myself. I was going to tell him that I loved him. I opened my eyes just before I opened my mouth, and what I saw rendered me silent. He looked disgusted and shocked. As he pulled back, my legs flopped away from him. I suddenly realized how cold it was inside the car. "You're a sex maniac!" he said. At that moment I felt like I had been struck. I had thought we were in this together. Why was he masturbating me if he didn't want to give me pleasure? Was a certain amount of pleasure okay and any more than that sick? Was there a pleasure limit? I'd brought him to climax many times. Were only males entitled to orgasm?

The phrase "double standard" wasn't part of my lexicon at that time, but it sure was part of my life. If I had thought that judgment ended at the confessional or with my mother's generation, I was proven wrong. I can't remember anything else that happened that night. John and I stayed together for a couple of years, but I never had an orgasm with him again. In fact, I didn't have another one until I was nineteen and met the man who would change my life.

5.

no magic: george

....

"**L**ook, I just want to be able to have sex. How is this supposed to help?" My second session with George wasn't going any better than the first had two weeks earlier. I was teaching him how to do Kegel exercises and after only one round of practice he stopped. When I was in mid-inhale, demonstrating the exercise, I opened my eyes to find him smirking at me.

"Kegels can help you feel arousal more intensely and give you greater control over the PC muscle. Both will help you to build up the time you can sustain an erection and defer orgasm," I said. I tried to keep my tone even. Getting irritated wouldn't help. George's eyes narrowed with anger, as if I had just insulted him.

It was 1974 and George, at fifty-two, had come to see me for premature ejaculation. He had a wife and a mistress and he could have sex with neither because he couldn't maintain an erection for more than a few minutes. Because he couldn't talk about it, his mistress was drifting away and he swore he could feel his wife losing respect for him. Two people to have sex with and not one to talk to, I thought.

Madelyn, George's therapist, had warned me that he was cantankerous. That alone I could have dealt with. She had hoped that doing hands-on work would help because George resisted nearly everything she tried with him.

The real problem, I was now convinced, wasn't that he was a curmudgeon. It was that he expected miracles and didn't want to put effort toward resolving the issue he faced. He wanted his problem to simply go away without investing any time or energy in building new skills, improving communication, or reimagining his sex life. Well, there is no magic potion, no open sesame, for overcoming sexual problems. It takes work and a commitment to change.

"George, there are solutions to your problem, but you have to be willing to learn some new skills and to communicate better. That takes time."

He rested his broad forehead in both hands and let out a sigh.

It wasn't anything I hadn't told him in our first session, when I should have concluded that I could not help George. For most of our two hours together he was silent, and when I asked him a question his answer came in monosyllables, apart from one notable exception. I'd tried to talk to him about how sexuality changes as we age. Big mistake. He insisted he still had the prowess of a twenty-two-year-old. That was when he let me know that as a kid growing up in Indiana he had been awarded medals for being the fastest runner on his track team. In his twenties he had won marathons and he still did daily long-distances runs. He was faster and stronger than his twenty-five-year-old son. "Nothing's changed with me," he said.

"How did you feel about our first session?" I asked George.

"It was okay."

"Did you find anything helpful?

"Not really."

"What were you hoping to get out of it?"

He glared at me.

"Let's discuss what we're going to explore today."

I explained that we would try Sensual Touch again, just like the first session, only this time, after I explored him, he would touch me.

"I don't need another massage."

"George, I know you're frustrated, but if you want help, you have to go through this process. It's not going to happen instantly."

"I know, that's what you've said."

By now I was struggling to keep my voice and expressions neutral. I reminded myself to be compassionate, but I was also wondering why George was here. He didn't seem to have faith in me or in surrogacy work. I told myself to see him as a challenge. Maybe I could convince him to open his mind to some of the exercises and understand that if he wanted a different result he had to try to change his behavior and his way of thinking.

We went to the bedroom and undressed. When George flung his tan suede coat on the chair next to the bed I was reminded of how broad his shoulders were. It landed spread out, arms hanging over the sides of the chair. George didn't have a thimbleful of fat any-where on his triangle-shaped body. His brown hair was thinning a little on top. He combed it back, so that a spray of it hovered slightly above his head.

The December cold had chilled the air in the bedroom, so I turned up the heat. I asked George to tell me if it got too warm. Then I pulled back the bedspread and invited him into bed.

I got in next to him. He stretched his arms over his head so his ribs jutted out.

I asked George to take some deep breaths.

He made a sniffing sound, accompanied by a single sharp inhale.

"And then let that breath out."

He blew out as though he were blowing up a balloon.

He stopped and stared at me with unvarnished contempt—a look I had seen on the faces of many of the adults I'd known in my younger life. It touched a raw nerve, and only a few years ear-lier it probably would have made me feel exposed, affirming my deeply held conviction that I was a horrible person. Now, it made me angry, though I willed myself to contain my emotions and to remain professional.

I asked him to mentally scan his body from head to toe to detect and relieve any tension.

"Focus on your eyes. Do you feel any tension there?"

No answer.

"How about around your mouth?"

Silence.

"I notice some tension in your jaw. Can you release it?"

George still said nothing. His eyes looked like stones, and his body was as tight as a compressed spring.

Finally he said, "This is a joke. You really get paid for this? Again, how is this supposed to help?"

That was it. I had tried my best to work with George, but now I was done.

"It won't help, George. It won't help because you're not willing to try. I'm not sure why you came here, but I think it's clear that you're not ready to put in the effort."

I stood up, put on the robe that lay over my chair, and told George to get dressed. He swung his legs over the side of the bed, his big feet landing on the floor with a thud. He pulled the leg of his pants off of the chair and all of his clothes toppled down. He glanced at me to see if I had noticed it and then quickly looked away when he realized I had. He thrust both legs into his trousers, put on his pullover, wedged his feet in his socks and shoes, and grabbed his coat.

I followed him down the hall to make sure he was on his way out.

When he reached the foyer, he turned to me and said, "I wouldn't take a woman like you anywhere but a McDonald's," and then threw the door open.

George's attitude reminded me of the binary attitude that pervaded my childhood. There were two kinds of women: the nice girls and the whores. I had hoped that I had left that in my past. Still, I have to admit he also made me doubt my own performance. If I were a better surrogate would I have been able to help him? Could I have done more to inspire him to change?

After I had cooled down a bit I called George's therapist and explained what had happened. "I did my best," I said to Madelyn, "but I just couldn't get through to him."

"Cheryl, we can't help everyone who comes to us," Madelyn replied.

At this early stage in my career, just a year into it, it was important for me to hear this. I felt so passionately about surrogacy work and I wanted to believe that I could help everyone who came to see me. Even in those early days, I had seen clients transformed by this work. And it wasn't only the client who benefitted. The process of becoming a surrogate had changed how I saw myself and my potential. For a moment, the work with George had opened up that well of self-doubt that I'd worked hard to fill.

6.

no virgin mary

By the time I was a senior in high school, I had visited just about every Catholic parish in Salem and a few outside of it. I made the rounds and juggled priests, usually with my friends Marcie and Lisa. It was my way of avoiding confessing the same sins to the same priest and receiving the same reaction every Saturday. As I cycled through different parishes I thought I could maybe convince the priests (and perhaps even myself) that I wasn't a serial sinner.

One cold October morning I walked the tree-lined route to St. Mary's with Marcie and Lisa. My legs felt rubbery and my stomach was doing back flips. I was also unusually quiet. "What's wrong?" Marcie asked. "Oh nothing, just tired," I answered. In reality, I was panicked. I was about to confess a mortal sin—again. I was thumbing my nose at God's law. At least with Bill, I could tell myself that I was sinning for love. God might not forgive that, but maybe he'd show some mercy because of it. Intimacy with John was just for pleasure.

I was trading my soul for a good time in the backseat of a Dodge on Kernwood Road. What kind of a person was I?

I had a few brief moments of relief when I walked into St. Mary's and felt a welcome rush of heat, but my anxiety quickly returned and soon I was sweating. The earthy scent of incense made me feel even queasier. I tried to remind myself that afterward my friends and I would head over to Forest River Park, meet up with other friends, and the fun would start. We would spend hours laughing and gabbing. C'mon. Calm down, I told myself.

I sat in the confessional and tried to settle down. A few seconds later the priest entered the other side of the booth. Through the iron lattice I could see his cheek, which looked yellowish in the dim light. "Forgive me, Father, for I have sinned. It has been one week since my last confession." I started describing some venial sins: To spare her feelings, I had told my cousin that I liked her new hairstyle, when I really didn't. I had felt envious of a friend who was going off to college in New York City. I had lied to my mother. Then, it was time for the big one. I admitted to having sex with my boyfriend.

The priest had been silent up until then, and had he remained so, I probably would have seen him—or one of his counterparts—the same time next week. Instead, he said, "It's girls like you who ruin young boys' lives." Suddenly my fear turned to anger. In that single moment, all my timid questioning, all my quiet skepticism, finally gave way to rage. I hardly had to cajole John into having sex. Perhaps I was a sinner, but was he really a victim? Wasn't he equally culpable? "What about my life, Father?" I asked. "Twelve Our Fathers and nine Hail Marys" was his only response. I left the church that day without saying a single prayer and I never returned to confession.

I continued to go to Mass every Sunday with my family. It would have been nice if all of my shame and guilt evaporated when I decided to stop going to confession, but it didn't. I still took communion. Yet another sin. When the priest placed the wafer on my tongue I had trouble swallowing it. I was submerging the symbol of the most holy and pure into the rot inside of me. Without confession, my guilt now multiplied. And yet, I had broken free from a dogma that I knew was irrational, unfair, and unkind. I had started to form a new identity apart from the Church and it was both exciting and frightening. That's not to say that my struggle was over. I still vacillated between anger and fear, reason and belief.

In 1962, my last year of high school finally arrived. What I was going to do for a career was not a matter of much concern for my family. My brothers had to go to college because they were future breadwinners and a solid education would give them an edge in the job market. My father, in particular, thought spending money on higher education for me made about as much sense as buying a car for our cat. True, my poor grades in grammar school had kept me out of the classical, or college-prep, track in high school. But even if they hadn't, I had no reason to believe that a college career would have been encouraged or funded. A girl like me, it seemed, should be satisfied just to find a husband who could provide for her and the kids she would soon bear.

My guidance counselor, Mrs. Russo, was the first one to mention Bay State Academy in Boston to me. Bay State offered a two-year secretarial program that taught typing, shorthand, and other skills that I could parlay into an office job, one of my few employment possibilities. When I discussed it with my parents, my dad scoffed. What did I need more schooling for? For her part, my mother became a surprising ally. She insisted, against my father's strident objections, that he would fork over the money for me to start Bay State in the fall. So, as my last year of high school wound down, I got ready to go to what would be the closest thing to a college I would get near for quite awhile.

Bay State Academy was actually a great experience for me. I met women I liked and I learned some valuable skills. That's why, when it came time for the second year, I was disappointed when my father put his foot down and flat out refused to pay for it. "It's a waste of money," he declared. Especially now, since Dave Mallory at Kressler Engineering had a job opening that would be perfect for me. Dave was an old friend of my father's. He was the vice president at Kressler, a thriving structural engineering firm in Boston. I had learned enough at Bay State Academy to do the available job and to save my father a year of tuition. If he only knew who I would meet at Kressler and the path it would start me on, Dad would have happily written the check for my second year at Bay State.

&

At six-foot-two, Michael Cohen had a commanding presence, and when he swaggered through the Kressler office few people, regardless of where they sat on the corporate totem pole, failed to notice him. After his size, the first thing I noticed about Michael was his hands. They were long and delicate, yet strong. He was twenty-three, had flawless skin, dazzling blue eyes, and a deep voice that was so sexy it sometimes made my knees weak. He also had blond, wavy hair that he wore long—or at least what was considered long for the time. Michael was the "office boy," but if there was ever a misleading title that was it. That his intellect and confidence soared above his position was apparent to everyone.

When he wasn't running errands for our bosses or printing blueprints, Michael sat in the desk next to mine. One Monday morning, when I asked him how his weekend was, he responded with, "Great, I fucked all weekend."

"Whaaaaaat?"

"Yeah, we just got up to eat."

Was this guy for real? No one—and I mean no one—in my world talked about sex that openly. His comment left my eyes wide open and my jaw hanging. I must have looked silly, but it didn't faze him. He then asked me about my weekend, but I was dumbfounded and couldn't respond.

Michael and I started eating lunch together regularly, and soon we were in an ongoing dialogue. He could ask me anything, even the most personal question, and not seem like he was prying. Never before had I had such straightforward discussions. We talked a lot about sex, but we also talked about movies, politics, books, his college courses, my family, his family, our dreams for the future, and everything else under the sun. Yet, if our conversations were forthright, they weren't always honest. At first I told him I was a virgin because I feared he would think less of me if he knew the truth.

Michael had been suspended from Boston University for taking tests for other students. When he was caught taking an exam for a business major, he was called before the disciplinary board. He defended himself by pointing out that the student who had hired him was a future captain of industry who had made a sound business decision by finding the best man for the job and hiring him. Needless to say, the board wasn't persuaded and slapped Michael with a one-year suspension.

Nothing about Michael was conventional. He kissed me before our first date. We were in the elevator descending to the ground floor for lunch when he reached out and gently pulled me to him. He planted the most sensuous kiss on me that I'd ever received. It was tender and erotic at once. There were never any half-measures with Michael. Everything was done with passion, and that kiss was no exception.

With Michael, I started to flourish. I grew out my hair and bought a new, sexy, Michael-approved wardrobe. He gave me a reading list and suddenly I realized I was smart and had insight into literature that none of my teachers had been able to evoke. We dabbled in marijuana and psychedelic drugs. Sexually, I explored even more. I had and gave oral sex for the first time with Michael, and I also had my first orgasm with intercourse. Just as important, I made love for the first time with the lights on, and I had conversations about what I liked and didn't. It was a time when life teemed with possibilities, and together we set out to explore them.

For Michael, most of what I had been taught about sex was barely worth taking seriously. "Ridiculous," he laughed when I told him about the prohibition against masturbation and other Catholic dogma that had passed for sex education in my childhood. "It's about control. Keeping you scared and ashamed is how they control you," he declared. He even seemed angry that I had been subjected to so much hurtful misinformation. Could it be that the problem really wasn't with me, but with the doctrine?

For the first time in my life I had the opportunity to have open, nonjudgmental, and genuinely frank discussions about sex. Michael approached sex from a secular perspective that was new to me. Now, not only could I challenge what I had been taught, but I could also arrive at alternative opinions and ideas that actually made sense to me. One night, long after I had come clean about my sexual past, I told Michael about my last experience in the confessional. "Idiotic," he sniffed. "Why do they have such a hang-up about virginity? It makes no sense," he added.

I explained how I believed God was watching as I wantonly dismissed the rules, and my fear that when I died, he would act. Michael scoffed at this. After all, he wasn't Catholic. He was Jewish. At the time I had no idea what that actually meant. All I knew was that he didn't seem to think of God as some kind of cruel schoolmaster.

Only weeks into our relationship, Michael and I maintained separate addresses on paper only. I was nineteen and shared an apartment with two other women in Boston, but I spent most nights at Michael's place. My parents knew about Michael and we had what I considered to be an unspoken agreement to avoid the question of whether or not we were sleeping together. They didn't ask and I didn't tell.

Early one morning when I was at Michael's apartment the phone rang. I still had an hour before I had to get up for work and I considered not answering, but around the fifth ring it was clear that the caller wasn't going away. Michael covered his head with his pillow. Half-asleep, I grabbed the receiver.

"We have to talk," my father said.

"Dad?"

"You have to come home this weekend."

"How did you get this number?"

"He's in the book. You have to come home this weekend. We need to talk."

I had the sinking feeling that our unspoken agreement had just come to an abrupt end.

That weekend as I took the bus to my parents' house, I had a feeling familiar to what I'd experienced on those Saturday morning treks to the confessional.

I had to steady myself before I opened the front door.

"Let's talk in the den," my father said.

This can't be good, I thought, as I followed him. What he said next left me reeling.

"It's obvious you're no Virgin Mary. I know what you've been up to with your boyfriend."

I gulped. I felt like I had just been slapped in the face. Then it got worse.

"You might as well marry him because no decent man would have you now."

I started crying. I was speechless. My father had essentially deemed me damaged goods.

That night, Michael and I spent hours talking. The guilt and shame had been heaped back on me in full force. First, my priest tells me that I'm the kind of girl who ruins young boys' lives, and now this. It seemed I couldn't escape judgment, even if I had fooled myself into believing that I had. When I told Michael about what my father had said, his response was predictable and comforting. "Your father's living in prehistoric times. No 'decent' man would care if you're a virgin or not."

I tried to explain to him again how the Church had turned me against myself, how it had made me feel shame for having any interest in sex. When I was done talking, he said something so lucid, so simple, and that still remains profoundly true to me today. "There is no God who is less compassionate than you." I had never thought of God as compassionate, but I realized then that I could no longer believe in one who wasn't.

7.

better late than never: larry

....

When, exactly, is the optimal time to lose your virginity is a question I can't answer. For my parents and the Church it was only after you had said "I do." At fourteen, I felt tremendous guilt for having sex for the first time with Bill. Mark O'Brien was ashamed to find himself a virgin at thirty-six. Just what age is the right age depends on so many factors I doubt even an army of relevant professionals could arrive at a definitive answer. I do know, however, that my client who lost his virginity with me in 2005 was decades past the age when most of us consider it normal to first have sex.

"Seventy?" I asked Carol, a local therapist who sometimes sent clients to me. "Seventy. He just celebrated his birthday," she answered. Carol smiled and took a sip of coffee. We were sitting in a café around the corner from her office when she told me about Larry. By this time I had been a surrogate for roughly three decades, and working with septuagenarians wasn't new for me. I did a double take not because of his age, but because of the issue he was dealing with: Larry was a seventy-year-old virgin.

"Wow. Pretty brave of him to tackle this now," I said.

"So I guess I'll send him your way?" Carol replied.

A few days later Larry called and scheduled his first appointment with me.

He had a full head of straw-colored hair and a grey-flecked beard. His eyes were so dark that the pupil and the iris were indistinguishable. At seventy, he continued to work at the engineering firm he had helped to start nearly forty years earlier. He couldn't remember a time in his career when he worked fewer than fifty hours a week.

Even though it was January, he wasn't wearing a coat. When I asked if he was warm enough he said that January in the Bay Area was like the Caribbean compared to the Chicago winters he had grown up with. "They weatherproofed me for life," he added. I smiled and motioned for him to sit down on my office sofa.

Larry was articulate and insightful, and he had thought a great deal about how his upbringing had shaped his life. He was an only child raised by parents in a miserable marriage. His mother devoted nearly all of her energy and attention to Larry. "My mother sacrificed everything for me," he said, "and she demanded a lot of me in return." Academic achievement was everything. While she would never admit it, Larry had believed for a long time his mother expected him to support her after he had completed the advanced degree that would land him a high-paying job.

He knew from an early age that his mother felt trapped. She had little education and at the time there were few career options for women, so she stayed with his father, the breadwinner of the family. She insisted that socializing and dating were luxuries Larry could indulge in later, after critical goals had been achieved and his economic status secured. "Frivolous. That's what my mother called any extracurricular activity, including dating," he said. "She thought if I got a good education and then a good job, everything else would just fall into place. It made me think that affection was some kind of prize you earned for accomplishing stuff, not something you just got for being you." There was a directness that bordered on urgency in how he talked, and, unlike many other clients, I had to do very little to ease his history out of him. Larry wasn't only ready to have sex, he was ready to tell his story.

When Larry finally suspected he had achieved enough to merit a relationship, he was already in his thirties and so self-conscious and anxious about his lack of experience that his attempts at intimacy fell flat. He recounted one particularly painful story about a woman he dated for a brief time. Kathleen was attractive, funny, and smart and he fantasized about a future with her. "I dreamed of coming home to her every day, of her face lighting up when I walked through the door, of her . . . wanting me," he said. When Kathleen started to talk about past relationships, however, Larry quickly changed the subject to one he was more comfortable with. His level of education gave him plenty of other topics to choose from, and he became what he called a "master of the creative segue," a skill he found useful whenever a conversation shifted to talk of relationships.

Their third date was the last for Larry and Kathleen, and the last ever for Larry. He remembered that she wore a tight pink dress and he felt aroused from the moment he saw her that night. As he sat across the table from her at dinner, he felt himself getting hard and he started to panic. He got so jittery he spilled his glass of wine. "In my mind I tried to talk myself down and focus on the conversation as much as I could, especially since I could see my anxiety was making her nervous," he said. As dinner went on he relaxed and by the end they were feeling close enough for Kathleen to ask him to continue on to her apartment.

They walked hand in hand and there were moments when Larry thought this might be the night that ushered him into a world it seemed every other adult but he had entered already. "I kept thinking that the next day I would wake up a different person—a normal person," he said. After a quick drink, Kathleen led Larry into her bedroom. They sat on the bed and started kissing, or tried to. When

Kathleen pressed her lips to his, Larry's anxiety escalated to panic. "I felt like I was being speared through my chest and I could feel my stomach convulsing," he said. He got up, stammered good night to a confused Kathleen, and left. He bolted down the two sets of stairs that led to her apartment and continued to run until he could barely breathe. "I literally ran away," he said. He looked down at his shoes, and I could hear him saying "okay, okay, okay" softly as he tried to pull back from crying.

"It's very brave of you to come here, and you're not alone in your anxiety," I said.

He leaned back in his chair with his eyes closed for a few seconds and then told me he didn't want to die without having sex.

Larry had run away from so much that night and it was heart-breaking to think of someone going through his whole life without tasting the joy and intimacy of sex and relationships. While he may have stayed in it longer than most, Larry was in a vicious circle that traps and paralyzes too many of us. He was anxious and fearful because of his lack of experience. This led him to avoid sex and kept him inexperienced, which compounded his anxiety, which, in turn, made him more averse to sex and intimacy. The sad outcome of all of this was the grinding loneliness Larry lived with for nearly all of his seventy years.

We talked for a little while longer. I told him about the surrogacy process and reassured him that his fear was not uncommon and that we would go at a pace that was comfortable for him.

When we got to the bedroom, I closed the blinds, drew back the beige top sheet on my bed, and we both undressed. We lay down on our backs next to each other and I asked Larry if he was comfortable. He wanted to trade sides with me.

Larry was wide-eyed and a film of sweat covered his forehead.

"It's natural to feel anxious at this stage. It's why I always start by teaching some relaxation exercises," I said.

I asked Larry to put his hand on his abdomen and to start breathing deeply enough that he could see his hand rise and fall with each breath. I joined him, and we lay beside each other inhaling and exhaling for a couple of minutes.

"Now, let's check in with your body so you can free any tightness in it," I said.

I asked Larry to close his eyes and bring his mind to the top of his head. "In your mind's eye see the top of your head. Then feel where your head meets your neck. If you're holding any tension in the back of your neck, drop your chin slightly and see if that makes it more comfortable. As I walk you through your body, make any adjustments you need to be more at ease.

"Now be aware of your shoulders and your shoulder blades and the space between them. Be aware of the contact they make with the bed. Notice where your shoulders and your arms connect. Come down your upper arms, into your elbows, forearms, wrists, and hands. Take slow, deep breaths. Then come back to your chest. Be aware of your pectorals. Then your abdomen."

We continued to drift down his body.

When we reached his feet, I asked him to wiggle his toes and then let them relax.

Larry and I took a few more breaths together.

"How do you feel now?" I asked.

"Better. More fluid, not as tight," he said.

We moved on to Spoon Breathing. Larry lay on his side and I nestled behind him. "Just take nice, easy, normal breaths," I said. I followed the rhythm of his breathing and soon we were breathing in and out together.

Spoon Breathing usually makes clients feel safe and nurtured, and I could feel Larry's body become ever looser as we snuggled together, breathing in unison.

I stayed in this position a few minutes longer than I normally would have. This was the first time Larry had been touched in a sensual way in decades. I knew he was frightened and I wanted him to have a sense of feeling secure and cared for.

After several minutes, Larry rolled over onto his abdomen and we began Sensual Touch. I started at Larry's feet. They were bony and he had thick toenails. I cradled his feet in my hands and made circles around the arches and heels.

Larry's legs were covered in light brown hair and, as I inched my palms up them, I could feel the muscles releasing under my hands. The tightness dissipated just as quickly in his butt and back and neck. Larry's body was starved for touch. When I got to the crown of his head, I started back down to his toes. His skin had a creamy tone, and, despite his age, he didn't have many wrinkles.

I moved my hands gradually down and asked him to take a deep breath when I got to his feet. I squeezed his feet gently, and when he exhaled I let them go. Then I said, "When you're ready, turn over."

Larry had an erection and he reflexively covered it with his hand.

"It's okay. It's a natural response," I said

He slowly moved his hand away.

I went up his body. When I got to his penis, I glided my finger over it and made my way up his groin and abdomen. I reached the top of his head and then started back down.

When we were finished with Sensual Touch, I asked Larry how he felt. "Like I've had a glass of ice water after being in the desert," he said.

Over the next four sessions, Larry and I engaged in a number of exercises designed to help him become less anxious, more at peace with his body, and better able to express himself verbally and physically. As with Mark and most of my other clients, we had to address not just Larry's particular sexual issue, but the emotions that shadowed it. He was surprised to learn that many men, no matter how experienced, occasionally feel anxious and tentative in sexual situations. He was also surprised to learn that being over fifty and sexually unfulfilled wasn't an aberration.

I was careful to take it slow with Larry. Touch was so unfamiliar to him and he had built up so much anxiety from his years of unhappy abstinence that it took some time for him to connect with his body. There were moments when Larry could barely believe he was finally engaging with a woman in a sexual way. It was no surprise that he often felt confused and tentative when we explored each other. Letting him gradually experience varieties of foreplay and slowly learn about my body helped Larry to feel more confident and at ease once he finally lost his virginity.

Larry's fifth session was scheduled for February 12, and one of the first things he said to me when we he arrived was, "I think this is going to be the first year I'm not miserable on Valentine's Day." It was time for Larry to finally have sex.

After checking in with him to see how he had been doing since our last visit, we headed to the bedroom and undressed. We lay down next to each other and did some relaxation exercises. I gently caressed down Larry's body and unrolled a condom over his hardening penis. I took it into my mouth and it quickly blossomed into a full erection.

We did some deep breathing to keep him where he was on the arousal scale. Then I climbed on top of him and slid him into me. I slowly moved up and down, and after a few minutes we rolled over so he was on top of me. He started thrusting his hips. Soon he had inadvertently slid out of me and I saw a spasm of panic cross his face. "It's okay," I said, "That happens. Sometimes you'll slip out." I grabbed a pillow and put it under my hips. "This usually helps," I said. "You're doing great. Try to not withdraw so far, but it's not a problem to guide your penis back into me if you do." I took Larry's penis in my hand and brought it to my vulva. "Okay, go ahead and push now," I said. Soon Larry was in me again, moving slowly in and out. "When this happens with a future partner, feel free to ask her to help you back in, or do it yourself—whichever is easier," I whispered in his ear.

He asked if he could kiss me, and when I said yes he lay flat on top of me, using his elbows for support and softly brought his lips to mine. He explored my mouth and my lips with his tongue. After a few minutes he lifted himself up and started thrusting again. His forehead was slick with sweat and a few drops fell onto my face. Then he shouted, came, and rested his head on my chest. I wrapped my arms around him. At seventy, Larry had lost his virginity.

I could see tears welling up in his eyes. This was a gratifying moment. I had helped this sensitive, smart, and kind man finally have one of the most fundamental and pleasurable human experiences. Larry's life had been full of accomplishments, but bereft of physical affection and intimacy. Together, we had changed that for him, and it was one of the most tender moments of my career.

I wanted to be sure Larry felt nurtured and cared for after his first time, so I suggested a round of Spoon Breathing and we shifted to our sides. After about our fourth cycle of breathing, Larry stopped and said, "This means so much to me." I gently pressed myself into him. "You know," he said, "I once learned there was a rumor going around about me being gay. I didn't try to correct it because being a virgin who's eligible for social security is more freakish than being a homosexual." Then he laughed a little and told me he had never admitted that to anyone.

It isn't unusual for clients to reveal things to me they keep hidden, even within the safety of their therapist's office. It is part of what makes surrogacy work fascinating and often beautiful. The surrogate's bedroom is a unique environment in which both professional and client are vulnerable. Being naked together is a powerful equalizer, and before any touch even occurs the mood can shift and intimacy can deepen so that people begin to talk more freely than they ever thought they would. Mostly, they share experiences that have had an impact on their lives, but about which they've always been too ashamed or embarrassed to reveal. Just saying them aloud can be liberating for some clients because suddenly they can gain a perspective few of us have when we hold tight to a secret.

8.

westward

· ·

"You're the devil!" my mother shrieked at Michael from across our living room. She stood behind the recliner as if she were trying to shield herself from him. My friend Marshasue, her boyfriend, Ronnie, and I all froze. Michael remained as loose-limbed and calm as ever. It was a warm Saturday in June and the four of us were heading out to Marblehead for a picnic. It occurred to me then that I should have bought a new can of Off! mosquito repellent instead of swinging by my parents' house to get the one I had there.

"What are you doing to my daughter?" my mother screamed.

"I'm not doing anything to her," Michael said in a cool voice.

"You're evil, evil incarnate."

"Mom, stop," I said, through a clenched jaw. "Let's go. Now," I added.

I turned to leave and the three others followed behind me.

"'Bye, Mrs. Theriault," Michael said before closing the front door.

I wanted to kick him. There was no need to make a bad situation worse.

I had hoped that the struggle with my parents was over, that they had resigned themselves to having a wayward daughter, and now they would gracefully recede and let me live my debauched life. If only.

Dave Mallory, my dad's friend at Kressler Engineering who had recommended me for the job, had talked to my parents about Michael. He told them that Michael was outspoken, hedonistic, contrarian, a rebel of the first order—all the things I loved about him. He let them know that I had latched on to a man who had no future, someone who was incapable of providing a stable life for me. Son-in-law material he was not.

Mallory also told my parents about a bet Michael had made with some of the other guys at work. Michael wagered that he could get me into bed, and one Friday when I showed up with an overnight bag he let them know that he would collect the following Monday. Maybe Dave was looking out for my best interests. That was a pretty crass thing to do, and when I learned about it I had one of the first inklings that Michael might not be as devoted to me as I wanted to believe he was. At the time I believed that Dave was threatened by Michael, whose intelligence and wit were widely admired at work. A few of the other executives had even talked about funding his return to college because they recognized that Michael could quickly become an asset to Kressler. Whatever his mix of motives, though, Dave had convinced my parents that I now shared a bed with Satan himself.

A few weeks after the confrontation in my parents' living room, Mom and Dad initiated what they must have thought of as a rescue mission when they showed up at my apartment one evening with my grandmother in tow. Michael and I were kissing on the couch when the doorbell rang and in walked the three of them. What the hell were they doing here?

For a moment we all stood in my cramped living room staring dumbly at one another. I looked at my grandmother. Later she told me that the only reason she came was to make sure that violence didn't erupt between my dad and Michael.

"Why are you here?" I finally asked.

"We're here to take you home," my father replied.

"Dad, I'm not going back home."

My father turned to Michael, as if he were the one he was arguing with, and said, "We know what you're up to. You've had my daughter practically living with you. If you want to live with her, you marry her."

"Would you buy a pair of shoes without trying them on first?" Michael retorted.

My father's eyes looked like they were going to pop out of their sockets. He lunged for Michael and I screamed, "Dad, no!" I tried to grab his arm, but he was moving so fast I clenched my fingers into an empty fist. "Robair," my grandmother yelled, reverting to the French pronunciation of his name. He and Michael stood barely an inch apart. Besides being half his age, Michael towered over my diminutive father. He could have clobbered him without breaking a sweat.

"You don't want to do this," Michael said, never raising his voice.

"C'mon on, Daddy," I said, and grabbed his elbow.

My father stepped back and I only let go when he had cleared striking distance from Michael.

"Let's go," my mother huffed, glaring at me.

If my parents thought they would intimidate me into leaving Michael, they were proven wrong, but that doesn't mean I wasn't shaken. My heart raced and my body felt paralyzed and ready to sprint at the same time.

I was mostly angry at my parents, but Michael's remark had stung too. Likening me to a pair of shoes wasn't exactly flattering. In fact, it was downright insulting. And to be so crass in front of my parents, even if they were treating him poorly. I loved the freedom—sexual and otherwise—that life with Michael offered, but I also wanted him to think of me as special, and when I thought of metaphors for that, a pair of shoes didn't come to mind. I let it go, though, because to me Michael represented a one-way ticket out of the provincial life. He was everything my family, the Church, and my teachers were not. My thinking was very black and white back then. If he was their opposite, it could only mean that he was all good because they were all bad. It would be a while before shades of grey became visible to me.

Later that night Michael and I made love and he seemed even more attentive than normal. He was a dream lover and sex could go on for hours. He was slow, sensual, and made me feel like I was the most desirable woman in the world. We mused about what we wanted for our future and for the first time we discussed leaving Boston. We talked as though my parents were done meddling, but they would make a final attempt to separate us, and this time my mother would take the lead.

ℂ

I never really thought of my parents as bigoted. Salem was a fairly diverse city and both my mother and father seemed to mingle easily with people of other creeds and ethnicities. Rose and Arthur Solomon were good friends of theirs. They went to the movies together, ate at each other's homes, and took weekend getaways as a foursome. It didn't matter that the Solomons were Jewish. Yet neither of my parents was happy that Michael was. Friendship was one thing, but when it came to dating and marriage, only Catholics were welcome. When I was older I acknowledged this for what it was—a kind of gentile bigotry. My parents would never have been overtly hostile to someone because of his or her race or religion, but when it came to marriage the lines were drawn.

Mom and Dad assumed that Michael's mother and father, Sadie and Julius, would be equally dismayed to learn that their son was shacking up with a religious interloper. If my parents couldn't sever us, perhaps Michael's could. A few weeks after their mortifying visit to my apartment, my mother put in a call to Michael's mother. She banked on her news being a bombshell, so she must have been pretty disappointed to find Sadie nonplussed by it.

Michael's parents grew very dear to me and they always treated me with warmth and kindness, but it turned out they had prejudices of their own. "We were just relieved you were white," Sadie later told me. Michael had dated Latino and African-American women in the past and their fear was that he would cross racial, not religious, lines.

Michael would turn out to be one of the most charismatic people I'd ever meet. He was always at the center of his social circle and everyone from frat boys to hipsters to ordinary Joes were drawn to him. He had an uncanny knack for divining psychological motivations and subtleties. He made nearly everyone feel that finally they had met someone who understood them. Often, he played the role of the philosopher of the group, the one who had the insights, who could detect subterranean truth and hold you spellbound as he eloquently unearthed it for you.

Michael had a regular table at Jack and Marion's Deli in Brookline, just outside of Boston, where he held court with his entourage, myself included. We drank soda, ate massive corned beef sandwiches, and talked, talked, talked. This was 1964. Society was in flux and young people like us were questioning everything. Michael spoke with a certainty and confidence that eluded the rest of us. We had questions; he had answers.

More than once someone in his throng of admirers reminded me of how lucky I was to be his girlfriend. I was lucky. I never fully understood what Michael, who could have had any woman, saw in me. I knew that my success in landing two popular high school boys had to do with my personality and social intelligence, but this was Michael. He was a bon vivant who oozed sophistication and charisma. I knew I was out of his league, intellectually and physically. We were in Boston, surrounded by pretty college coeds. Of course, Michael had a reason for picking me, and one night as we lay in bed he revealed it. "You would be a great mother. I know you love fiercely. You're like a lioness and you'll protect the ones you love."

So, Michael wanted to have kids with me? Maybe this meant I was special.

◯

My mother, meanwhile, was relentless about breaking up Michael
and me. Having exhausted all of her other options, she kicked off a
campaign of near constant cajoling and nagging. She called me several times a day and wrote me letters besieging me to come home
and get back on the right track—as if I had ever been on it. Finally,
to get some relief from her, I agreed to return home for a year. She
knew I would still see Michael—I made that clear—but she desperately hoped that not living with him would cool the relationship and
make me realize that what I really wanted was a nice Catholic boy and
a suburban future. I still went into Boston to work and for the first
week I managed to come home every night. But as week number two
began, I pushed back and spent the night at Michael's. Then I stayed
another night. Soon Michael and I decided it was time to jettison my
parents for good and put an end to my exile to Salem. We would make
it official and get married, and we would do it soon.

When I told my parents about the engagement they were, not sur-
prisingly, livid. My mother squawked about boycotting the wedding;
my father sulked. For my part, I started going home a few nights a
week. Why not give them that since in less than a month I would be
Michael's wife and they would lose all authority over me?

Cantor Hammerman, a neighbor of Michael's parents, agreed to
perform the ceremony on one condition: that I was not pregnant.
Despite some close calls, I wasn't, so we decided to get married on
August 22, 1964, nine months after we met, in a small ceremony
in Cantor Hammerman's living room. In those days, especially for
women, marriage made you an adult. It didn't matter that I wasn't yet
out of my teens. In a short time I would officially be grown up and
beyond my parents' control.

I was thrilled and scared at the same time. On the night before the
wedding, sitting in my bedroom at my parents' house, it really hit
me that my life was about to change drastically. I looked around the
room that had never really been mine. The crocheted ecru bedspread,

the curtains with bluebonnets embroidered on them, the dressing table with the big oval mirror, the gilded brush and comb set that lay on it—all had been my mother's choices. She created the bedroom that she had wished for as a little girl and that even in my late teens I wasn't allowed to change. Nearly every day my mother made my bed and straightened up my room. If she needed to open my dresser drawers to put away laundry or rifle through my desk to find a roll of Scotch tape or a pair of scissors, she did it with no thought to my privacy. Worse, I was never allowed to close my door, and although Mom never explained why, I'm pretty sure this was a precaution against that evil of evils: masturbation. We may have called it my room, but it never was in any meaningful sense. Really, it belonged to my mother. I wanted out. I was desperate to get out, so why did I feel so much grief when I looked around at the frilly room my mother had made?

"Don't cry. Don't cry. You'll smudge your mascara," said my friend Lisa, who was my maid of honor, as we drove to Michael's parents the morning of the wedding. I was crying because I was sad and because I was ecstatic. My emotions danced about, ricocheting from high to low, a discordant combination of melancholy and elation.

When we arrived at Michael's parents' house, Michael was out running a few last-minute errands. Lisa carried in the simple white frock my grandmother had helped me pick out and I held my veil and satin pumps. When Sadie and Julius came to the door, they looked more serious than I had ever seen them. Sadie pressed a cookie into Lisa's hand and asked if she wouldn't mind ironing a table cloth they planned to use for the buffet. Then they led me into the living room and we sat on the couch.

"Cheryl, you know how much we like you . . . " Sadie began.

"That's why we have to have this talk," Julius continued.

"Michael will not provide for you. He's just not capable of building a stable life for a family. And if you have children, Sadie and I won't help you financially," Julius said.

If this declaration had been delivered differently I might have felt hurt, but Julius spoke with such genuine concern that I couldn't take it as anything other than a sincere attempt to protect me.

"I would never expect you to," I answered, perhaps too breezily.

"How old are you?" Julius asked.

"Nineteen. Old enough to know what I want," I answered.

"We hope so," Sadie said.

Despite my mother's threats, she attended the ceremony with my father, brothers, grandmother, and a few other family members. If my parents weren't joyous, they weren't disruptive either. All in all, the wedding was a simple and pleasant affair. Cantor Hammerman performed a civil ceremony that was free of any religious rituals. After we said our "I do's," the guests, who numbered around twenty, retreated to Michael's parents' house next door and mingled over corned beef, pastrami, coleslaw, rye bread, and other sumptuous deli food. We sipped champagne and Michael's best man, Jerome, made a toast wishing us a lifetime of happiness together. Even my parents raised their glasses.

⅍

Michael and I settled in Beacon Hill, a tony neighborhood in Boston. We rented a little one bedroom in an old brick building that had been sectioned into apartments. It had a small balcony with French doors leading onto it, and on warm nights we left them open. We turned our apartment into the go-to place for our social circle.

I soon left my job at Kressler because I got pregnant. A month into our marriage I missed a period. I went to the doctor, took a urine test, and learned I was expecting. Michael took a decent-paying job at the post office, which came with health benefits so that the cost of prenatal care and delivery would be covered.

If our financial status didn't worry me, what did was my ability to be a good mother. After all, I didn't have much of a role model. From the time I was very young, I believed my mother didn't like me. At first it hurt and I pined for her love and affection. Anger came later, but now I felt almost completely alienated from her. Would my child feel the same about me? Would I give her or him reason to? What if I was unable to love this child? I was terrified that I would repeat my mother's mistakes.

At Michael's suggestion, I started seeing a therapist once a week. It turned out to be the best thing I could have done for myself and my family. In therapy I was able to start the process of working through a lot of the anger, resentment, and guilt that lingered from my childhood. I gained the insight and confidence to be the kind of mother I wanted to be. As my child grew inside me, I knew I would love him or her, and that I would be the sensitive, caring mother I longed for, even then.

When I gave birth to our beautiful little Jessica in June of 1965, I knew that I would prove Michael's instincts about me to be true. I also knew that the relationship I had with her would be nothing like the one I struggled through with my mother.

Michael was everything I could have wanted in a father for my child. He was tender, caring, and sensitive to Jessica. Unlike so many other men of his generation, he eagerly became a full partner in parenting. He changed her diapers, scooped her up when she cried, and played with her. At night he turned on slow music, took her in his arms, and rocked her until she fell asleep. Before she could walk, Jessica had heard The Beatles, Donovan, The Grateful Dead, Joan Baez, and others in the pantheon of sixties rock and folk music. The Beach Boys' "Surfer Girl" was her favorite song and when Michael played it she would coo and smile and within minutes her eyelids would droop.

When Jessica was two-and-a-half and I was pregnant for the second time, Michael decided to return to college to get his bachelor's degree in education. Maybe having a child to nurture reminded him of what he had set out to become when he started at Boston University. Michael wanted to be a teacher and for him that meant something very particular. It meant being a mentor, someone who would teach kids not just facts, but how to think critically. He would inspire them to be their most thoughtful, creative selves and show them they could achieve anything they set their minds to.

In 1966, Michael enrolled in Boston State College. His mother was the secretary to the Dean of Admissions and she filed his paperwork for him and helped him get his credits transferred from Boston University. He left the post office job and took part-time work at the deli we frequented before we were married. He appealed to his parents for help and, despite their pre-wedding admonition, they agreed to assist us financially.

Michael also started working a night job in the cafeteria at Beth Israel Hospital. He left at 5:00 PM and returned home at around one in the morning. The job consisted of washing dishes and making breakfast porridge by the ton for the inpatients. He was instantly bored with it so, in typical Michael fashion, he found other outlets for his intelligence. He spent hours playing poker with the doctors and amassed a tidy sum from his winnings. He also returned to taking tests for college students whose ambition outstripped their integrity.

This reinforced something I had always thought about Michael. I knew he would never be a "straight" guy with a corporate job and a typical middle-class life, but I believed he would still be successful. Success for him—and, by default, me—would just look different from what our parents and mainstream society imagined.

Michael had no interest in being Ward Cleaver, and June made me want to wretch. Our future would be bright and it would be ours. We would make it what we wanted, not what we were supposed to want. That's why I brushed off Sadie and Julius's warnings. They were kind to be concerned, but they just didn't understand Michael.

⟢

Becoming parents didn't slow Michael and me down in the bedroom, but his new schedule did mean we had to carve out other times for sex. Even when it was only Jessica, I timed naps to coincide with Michael's arrival home from school and, with the vigor of two healthy twenty-somethings, our sex life continued unabated.

Our easy domestic routine held up until around June. That's when Michael suggested that I take Jessica out of town to my friends

Marshasue's and her husband Ron's farm in New Hampshire for a couple of weeks. Finals were just around the corner and he claimed he wanted some time to study without distraction. By this time I was almost seven months pregnant with our son. I really didn't feel like traveling—and I was suspicious.

Women were always fawning over Michael. Because of his unconventional attitude toward just about everything, I wasn't sure that he would consider having a wife a reason to resist them. He certainly was never jealous when other men came on to me, and no matter how happy I was about him, about us, I pretty much always had this gnawing feeling that I was not at all special to him, that I was just one of many who swirled around him vying for his attention. I wanted Michael to keep his free-spirited, alternative lifestyle and outlook, but I also wanted him to be so enamored of me that other women would appear unattractive by contrast. This wasn't about rules. It was about desire, and I wanted his desire to match mine. He wouldn't deny himself anything by being faithful to me because he wouldn't want anyone but me. I yearned for a comfy mix of bohemia and conventionality, one that would ensure my image as a rebel without inflaming my insecurities. Even at twenty-three I suspected real life was rarely so obliging.

But when Michael pressed for two weeks alone, I acquiesced. On a humid June morning I packed a suitcase for myself and Jessica, loaded our Volkswagen bug with a small zoo of stuffed animals, and headed north on I-93.

Michael and I talked every night. He told me how much he missed us and promised me he was preparing to ace his finals. I wasn't happy about being banished, but if it meant Michael's success at college then I would just have to suffer through a couple of weeks away from him.

Finally, Michael was done with his last exam and Jessica and I made the two-hour trip back to Boston.

"Daddy home?" Jessica asked as we turned onto our street.

"That's right, Sweetheart," I answered.

I parked the car, quickly freed Jessica from her car seat, and scooped her up. She giggled all the way to the front door.

Michael's grin lit up his face when he saw us. Jessica stretched out her arms and he pressed her to his chest and kissed her forehead. Then he planted a big smooch on me.

"I missed you two so much," he said.

"Not as much as we missed you. How did your last final go?"

"Nailed it. I'm expecting straight A's"

"Great!" I said and gave Michael another big kiss.

He went out to pick up burgers and fries for dinner. I unpacked and got reacquainted with my tiny home. It may not have been much, but it was all I needed. Besides, even the Taj Mahal wouldn't have been big enough to contain my love for my sweet little family.

Since Michael was now out of school, he went to work full-time at the deli. That his grades would be stellar was simply a given, and as the summer drew on it never occurred to me to ask about them. A few weeks later, I stood in my kitchen chopping carrots for the stew I was making for dinner. My belly was now so big that I had to fully extend my arms to reach the cutting board on the kitchen counter. My mind wandered as I mechanically chopped the carrots into rounds and then half-moons. Just as I was about to toss them into the pot on the stove the phone rang. It was Sadie.

"I just checked Michael's grades," she said.

Because of her position at the school Sadie had early access to final grades. Her voice sounded strained, but I couldn't imagine why.

"Yes?" I said.

"He dropped out of all of his classes. He got incompletes in every one."

I felt dizzy. I grabbed the back of one of the kitchen chairs and then lowered myself into it.

"What?" I stammered and then realized I did not want her to repeat herself. "How . . . how could that be?" I asked.

"I don't know, Cheryl. I was hoping you could explain it to me."

Well, I couldn't, and any explanation I could conjure up hurt too much for me to think about it for very long.

I was hurt, scared, and angry, and when Michael came home I lashed out.

"What the hell is going on?"

"What? What are you talking about?"

"I know, Michael. I know you didn't take your exams. Your mother told me. What were you doing those two weeks when you told me you were taking finals?"

Michael looked down at his shoes.

"Were you with another woman while Jessica and I were out of the picture for two weeks?"

"No. I was hanging out in the school cafeteria. I couldn't tell you, but I just didn't want to be in school anymore."

"So why did I need to leave?"

Michael said nothing.

I grabbed a lava lamp off an end table and slammed it down on the floor. The glass broke and the red-veined liquid expanded out on our hardwood floor like an amoeba.

Jessica started to cry.

"Mommy broke lamp," she said.

I picked her up and cuddled her.

"I'm sorry, Sweetheart. Mommy's sorry."

Jessica's tears were the only thing that could have stemmed my anger.

We ate dinner that night in total silence. I could now add guilt and humiliation to the list of toxic emotions coursing through me. I was stuck, and I knew it. What was I going to do? Return to my parents with my toddler and another one on the way? I could just hear the chorus of "I told you so."

And then there was the undeniable fact that I still loved Michael too much to walk away. Even if I had a warm, welcoming home waiting for my children and me in Salem, I would never go back to it. I loved Michael not just for who he was, but for how he made me see myself. I became the person I wanted to be with him. Around Michael, I was smart, funny, adventurous, and sexy—or at least that's how he made me feel. Michael listened to me. He wanted to hear what I had to say. He understood me. I had revealed myself to him and he had embraced me when many others had reproached me. I could no more leave Michael than go to the moon.

⌒

When early July came around, Michael announced that he wouldn't return to Boston State in the fall. I could feel the blood draining from my face as he explained that he was bored with the education program and that he needed more of a challenge. I would have been angry if I wasn't so scared—scared of losing Michael, scared that I wasn't enough for him, scared that he regretted marrying me. So, I simply said "okay."

A month later, in August 1968, our son, Eric, was born. Within four years I had left home, gotten married, and had two children. My life had radically changed, and soon it would take another major turn.

Michael and I had occasionally talked about leaving Boston for California. It was the heady days of the late 1960s and we both believed the world our kids were destined to inherit would scarcely resemble the one we knew. We were building a more just, freer, more tolerant society and it was just a matter of time before the transformation was complete. From our perspective, the epicenter of this new world was the San Francisco Bay Area. In the last few years some of our friends had headed there and we wondered what it would be like to join them. Sometimes they would call us from their apartment and hold the phone out the window so that we could hear the bustle of the street. "You've got to come to San Francisco. People smoke grass in the street here!" they would cry into the phone. In October 1968, we called our friends and asked if we could stay with them for a few weeks until we found our own place.

I so wished that moving to California would motivate Michael to do something more with his life. I hoped that he would hit his stride out there and discover what it was that would make him happy. I was excited about our new life. So many possibilities waited for us, I was sure. I was also scared as hell.

Michael earned some cash by taking an exam for a friend who wanted to get into a doctoral program and we emptied our savings account. After buying a Volkswagen camper we had a $1,000 left to start our new life, no small sum at that time. We lined the back of the camper with sleeping bags and crammed in Jessica's menagerie of stuffed animals, plenty of drawing paper and crayons, and enough books and toys to keep her occupied for the cross-country trip.

On the morning we left we stopped by some friends' houses to say goodbye and then drove to my parents' house. My mother was furious. She took our leaving as a personal affront, and when I hugged her she stiffened her body and kept her hands at her sides. My father had tears in his eyes, and when I turned to him he said, "Go ahead and leave. The next time you see me I'll be in my coffin." My father was a healthy forty-six-year-old, but at the time I wasn't thinking about how unrealistic and melodramatic this was. Peter, my fourteen-year-old brother, was crestfallen. He looked as though he was at a funeral. "I'll come back and you'll come visit me," I said to him, fighting back tears. Nanna was sad, but she said she wanted me to be happy. I promised I would call or write every week. I didn't stop sniffling until we were hours down the road and my sadness started to give way to excitement about the life that awaited us on the other coast.

Most of the trip was a lot of fun. We camped in KOA campgrounds. We stopped off at the Painted Desert and Petrified Forest and drove through cities like Oklahoma City and Santa Fe, which were so different from where I came from that they seemed nothing short of exotic. I nursed Eric, who started the trip just as he turned ten weeks, and three-year-old Jessica delighted in seeing the new sights that flashed before her every day. Everything was going smoothly, until about two weeks into our journey, when we were less than a 150 miles south of San Francisco.

The day started out like most days on the trip. We got up early, brushed our teeth with water from a canteen, and ate dry cereal for breakfast. I lay Eric in his car bed and Jessica lay on a sleeping bag in the back of the camper. Just as the sun started to rise we drove onto Highway 101. We traveled north for a few hours, the roadside scenery quickly unrolling alongside us. By 11:00 AM we were hungry and by noon we were famished, so just before we entered the town of Hollister we pulled into a diner. Including us there were probably ten people in the place, so we were served fast. We ordered club sandwiches for Michael and me and silver-dollar pancakes and a hot chocolate for Jessica. Michael and I each drained two cups of coffee and then asked the waitress to fill our thermos with more. Before 1:00 PM, we were back on the road. We all had full stomachs and Michael and I were caffeinated and ready to drive straight through the remaining two and a half hours to San Francisco. We would arrive at our new home before dinner.

As we pulled out of the diner parking lot, I took off my seat belt so I could nurse Eric on my right side. He stopped sucking for a moment and I look down. I wiped away a froth of milk bubbles that had collected around his mouth. I looked out the window and I saw a pickup truck with a camper built onto the bed barreling toward the interstate from a dirt road that led into it like a tributary. A brick-colored plume of dust kicked up behind it. They're going fast, I thought. Then we were close enough for me to see the rust on the fender. I saw the woman who was driving turn to the woman in the passenger seat, most of her profile obscured by her hair that hung loose. Isn't she going to stop?

Then an ear-shattering crash. Metal assaulting metal. Glass shattering into jagged shards and cascading to the pavement. The smell of rubber and the screech of tires moving with a new, uncontrollable momentum. I shouted, "Oh God!" All of us, in both vehicles, were trapped in the collision, slammed around by a force that gathered impossible strength in only seconds. We were upside down and Eric was on top of me, his mouth open and my chest covered in milk.

The horn wailed. Then we were right side up again. Smoke wandered out of the truck's hood like a ghost. Michael leapt out of the driver's seat, leaving his door open, and ran around to the passenger side. He helped Eric and me out of the camper. I screamed, "Jess . . . Get Jess." He ran to the back of the camper, ripped open the door, and extracted Jessica. Eric's face was blue. This isn't right. That's not how he should look. "No, no, no," I cried to Eric. Then he gasped and took a breath and the blue dissolved into pink as he screamed. I limped to the back of the camper and saw Jessica rubbing her sleepy eyes. "What happened?" she muttered.

Intense pain radiated from the top of my neck to below my shoulder blades. It kept me from standing up straight. The pickup truck had crashed into us, making our van summersault across the median, into the southbound lane. All four tires were blown and the rubber splayed out in black, jagged tongues. I heard sirens getting louder. Did this mean they were getting closer?

At the hospital they took X-rays of my back and found that I had three compression fractures between my shoulder blades and damage to the base of my neck. I realized later that Jessica had been protected by the truckload of stuffed animals we had packed for her. The impact tossed her around like a rag doll, but, fortunately, she careened from stuffed giraffe, to stuffed pig, to stuffed elephant. I was told that Eric was okay, but when he was around four he was treated for a neck problem that I attributed to the car wreck. Michael wore his seat belt and escaped with only a bruise on his foot. The doctor wrote me a prescription for Darvon and told me to take the next appointment I could find with an orthopedist.

Since our camper was totaled, Bobby, one of our friends in San Francisco, drove down to Hollister to pick us up. The five of us climbed into his van. Jessica sat on Michael's lap and Eric was in my arms for the two-and-a-half-hour trip north. Even the slightest bump or start made my neck scream, so I popped another Darvon. In retrospect, it seems like I should have asked the doctors if it was safe to keep nursing Eric while I took pain medication. Luckily it turned out that it was, but I didn't ask because at the time I assumed doctors were all-knowing and infallible.

We arrived at Bobby and Peggy's around 7:00 PM and I hobbled to bed. As I lay there staring up, the back of my head pressed flat against the mattress and the pillow flung to the floor, I worried about the toll my injuries might take on my sex life. What if I was hurt so badly that sex would be too painful, or what if I was no longer able to move enough to have it? I shook Michael awake.

"Huh . . . what . . . are you okay?" he said.

"I'm scared. I'm scared I won't be able to have sex again. So, let's try. Let's please try."

"Now? I thought you could barely move."

I turned over onto my side. A bolt of pain shot down my neck and into my back. I bit my cheek to keep from screaming.

"Okay, get behind me and, please, let's do it," I gasped.

Michael wedged himself up against me.

"Ow, oooh, ow," I whispered and my eyes misted.

"Are you okay?" Michael asked.

"Yes. Okay."

I turned my hips and lifted my leg a little so he could slide his penis into me.

"I'm afraid this will be the last time," I said.

"This isn't going to be the last time, Cheryl."

"I know, but if it is . . . "

"Cheryl, it's not the last time."

The next day I could barely move and Michael had to help me stand. Peggy found an orthopedist at a nearby hospital who could see me that day. Michael slipped a muumuu-style dress over my head and helped me to the car.

The orthopedist informed me that I had fractures in three of my vertebrae and a break at the base of my neck where it met my shoulders. Luckily, my spinal cord wasn't damaged. I felt so fortunate at that moment even though I would need to be in a brace for six months. The doctor disappeared for a few minutes and when he came back he held something that looked like a cross between a corset and a straightjacket. It was made of canvas and had rods that held it straight in the back. It closed in the front with Velcro-covered straps and was crisscrossed in the back with strings to tighten it. Normally, it would have covered my breasts and gone down to the base of my spine, but because I was still nursing Eric I couldn't have my breasts covered. The doctor fitted it just below them. I gasped in pain as he pulled the strings to tighten it to my body.

℘

Despite our inauspicious start, we did our best to get settled in the Bay Area. Michael began house-hunting and soon rented a bungalow across the bay in Berkeley. Julius sent us money, again. We still had several hundred dollars left from our original thousand and we used it to buy a 1954 Cadillac Coupe de Ville. Because it was yellow on the bottom and black on top, we dubbed it "the yellow submarine." After the accident, I wasn't taking any chances. The car may have been out of style, but it was safe. I felt like I was driving a moveable bunker and that's exactly what I wanted.

Michael was floundering and I was in no shape to hold a job, so we went on welfare. Between it and an occasional cash infusion from Julius and Sadie, we scraped by month to month. Our new home was across the street from an elementary school and I enrolled Jessica in kindergarten. I furnished our house mostly with Goodwill buys, reconnected with some other friends who had also gone west, and did my best to keep my spirits up.

The accident was terrifying and traumatic, but it eventually led me in one positive direction. As 1970 rolled around, I started to slowly recover my strength and mobility. I took yoga classes and did other exercises, but I was still inactive compared to my pre-accident days. I put on weight. Since my teenage years I'd always thought I was too fat, and it only got worse after the accident. This was the Twiggy era and curves had gone the way of car fins. I had never been clinically overweight, but as I was forced into a more sedentary lifestyle I felt out of shape. My new, fuller figure aggravated my body image issues and sometimes sent me into bouts of panic.

Every afternoon I waited on our front steps for Jessica to come home from school. She would come out in mid-afternoon, wave to me from across the street, and look both ways with her teacher and classmates. When it was clear to cross, she ran toward me with her arms flung out. It was the best time of my day, and it wasn't unusual for me to go out earlier than necessary to wait for her.

My schedule coincided with a neighbor's. She was a thickset woman with a heavy blonde braid that hung down to her waist. She'd always come by on her bike as I settled down on the steps with a book. As she cycled, her wide thighs pumped up and down and her large breasts jiggled, seemingly unrestrained by a bra. The rack on her bike was crammed with paintbrushes, colored pencils, and other art supplies, so I figured she was a student at the nearby art college. She looked to be around my age and we often smiled at each other.

One day as she pedaled slowly down the street I waved and said hello. She stopped and we started to chat.

"Are you an artist?" I asked.

"I'm taking classes at the art school and I also do some modeling," she said.

Modeling? The only models I'd seen were the wispy creatures who wore haute couture and haunted the pages of fashion magazines, the ones I wanted to look like.

This savvy, self-confident woman must have sensed my doubt. I hoped I hadn't offended her.

"I do nude modeling for the painting and sculpture students, and I'm more in demand than skinny women. They love all my curves and creases," she answered.

Suddenly I saw an opportunity. If she could model, so could I. I could earn some extra money and maybe even start to feel better about my body.

"How'd you get involved in that?" I asked.

"Oh, the school always needs models. It's a great way to earn some money, especially if you don't want a straight job."

I summoned up my courage and asked, "Do you think I could do it?"

"Sure. They'd be happy to have you." With a cobalt blue pencil she scrawled a phone number on the corner of a piece of drawing paper, tore it off, and handed it to me.

Within a year I was modeling regularly for students at local art schools and for a few full-fledged artists. I began to develop first an acceptance and then an appreciation of my body. Occasionally I saw flashes of excitement on the artists' faces, which surprised and delighted me. My body hadn't changed, but my perception of it sure was shifting. When I looked at their paintings and sketches of me, I saw them through the artists' eyes. The bulges that I thought were so awful actually began to look appealing.

Holding poses for lengthy periods also gave me plenty of time to think, and I started to reflect on the fluid nature of beauty. It was hard not to. I was coming to peace with a body that I had thought of as a misfortune for a long time.

For the first time in my young life, I started to think about how the notion of beauty isn't fixed, and how impossibly slippery the idea of the perfect body is. In those days, the waif was the ideal. A couple of decades earlier Marilyn Monroe could lay claim to the perfect figure. I did a little research and discovered Lillian Russell, a sex symbol in the late 1800s, who, at times, tipped the scale at two hundred pounds.

It was the beginning of a process of freeing myself from unrealistic, highly manufactured standards of beauty and perfection. Slowly, I started to realize that a perfect body probably can't be reliably defined, and even if it could, I didn't need perfection to feel good about the body that carried me through life.

I could not have known it then, but several years later this process would help me when I worked with one of the few women clients in my surrogacy career.

9.

past perfect: mary ann

As far as I could tell, Mary Ann's body was nearly perfect. She had long legs, a slim waist, and a stomach as flat as a baking sheet. Only her breasts, which were too big for her lithe frame, looked off and that was because they had been surgically enlarged. Jodie, Mary Ann's therapist, had described her as a stunning woman with body image issues, and when she walked into my office for our first session in 1988 that first part was obvious.

Up to this time I had only seen a few women clients. Most heterosexual women who seek the services of surrogates are referred to males, since so much of the work is about modeling a healthy sexual partnership. Mary Ann's difficulty in the bedroom sprung solely from a body image issue that her therapist believed I could help her address. As a surrogate, I looked forward to the challenge of working with a woman who struggled with an issue that affects so many of us. It would be a different dynamic and I would have to tailor the protocol to her needs, but I had a definite sense that I could help my new client.

When Jodie described Mary Ann to me, it seemed as though she were talking about a younger version of myself. Here was a woman who was both deeply insecure and profoundly uniformed about her body. I often thought about how much I would have benefited from the solid, nonjudgmental advice I hoped to share with Mary Ann.

At our first appointment, Mary Ann sat across from me on my office sofa. We chatted for a few moments before I brought up the concern that had brought her to see me.

"As you know, Jodie gave me some background on the issue that brings you here today. Can we start by talking a little about it?" I said.

"Okay," Mary Ann said.

I paused for a few seconds to see if she would continue. When she didn't I said, "Body image issues are very common, especially in women. I struggled with them for a long time."

"I'm not sure if it's a body image issue or if there is something really wrong with me."

"I understand from Jodie that you've been examined by your doctor and he doesn't see any abnormalities, so I think we can assume that this is a perception issue, rather than a medical one."

"So, you think it's normal."

"Do I think what's normal?"

"Having a vagina that's uneven."

I wasn't surprised to hear that this was at the root of her struggles. I could only assume she'd never seen another woman's labia. I did, however, want to understand why she assumed hers were abnormal. "Yes," I started, "but what you're talking about is not your vagina. It's your labia, and many women's are uneven."

Much of my work with Mary Ann would center on education, starting with anatomy. I explained to her that the vagina is internal and can only be seen with a speculum. The vulva, which includes the clitoral hood, clitoris, vestibule, labia minora, and labia majora, is the external part of the female genitalia.

Mary Ann was worried because the left side of her inner labia was longer than the right—or at least that is what she believed. She had never actually looked closely at her vulva, but when she felt it she could discern an asymmetry.

I planned to walk Mary Ann through a couple of exercises and show her some educational materials, but first I wanted to understand why she was so troubled by what she perceived as an imperfection. What did it really mean to her that her vulva was not "perfect?"

When I asked her about this she said it made her feel like she was secretly ugly to her husband and that it ate into her self-esteem to be anything short of physically flawless. Mary Ann prided herself on maintaining a beautiful body. At thirty-eight she had never had children. Regular tennis matches and Jazzercise had toned her muscles and sculpted the delicate curves in her five-foot, eight-inch frame. She obviously pegged a lot of her self-worth on what she looked like and I hoped that our work together would help to change that.

Surrogacy work takes many forms. It always includes a mix of education, exploration, and sexual play, but the balance between them shifts according to the client and his or her needs. For Mary Ann, my task would be to help her better understand that bodies— including vulvas—come in all different shapes and sizes, and that she was not at all abnormal or freakish. I wanted her to see that she comfortably fit into the spectrum of body types and to change her belief about being far outside of what was normal. I also hoped that I could help her dispense with Madison Avenue–generated standards of perfection, but that was, strictly speaking, beyond the scope of our work together.

Joania Blank's *Femalia* is a book that I often turn to in my work. It is a remarkable collection of color photographs that show the vulvas of thirty-two women. The differences between each one can be startling at first sight. Some of the models' vulvas are pink; others are brownish. Some labia are long, some are short; some are even and some are uneven.

I slid the volume off of my bookshelf and sat next to Mary Ann on the couch.

"Ready?" I asked.

I cracked it open and slowly we went through the thirty-two pictures.

"Wow," Mary Ann said as we thumbed through the pages. She asked me to hold on before passing over one photo of a woman whose inner labia hung down beyond the outer lips in two lush crescents.

"I never thought they could be that long," Mary Ann said.

We flipped through a few more photographs until we came to one that showed a woman with inner labia that hung about an inch longer on the right side than on the left.

"Is that normal—really?" Mary Ann asked.

"Absolutely. Lots of women have asymmetrical labia. It's just one of the many natural variants of female genitalia," I assured her.

"Really?"

"Really, and remember this is just a very small group of women. It doesn't represent all of the variety that's out there. It's no more unusual than having one foot that's slightly larger than the other. You probably wouldn't feel bad if that were the case, right?"

Mary Ann paused and looked down.

"No, but I thought that maybe I had damaged my vagi—vulva by masturbating."

"You haven't. I can assure you of that. It's just your unique shape and our goal is to help you become a little more comfortable with it."

She touched the photo with her fingertip as if to reassure herself of what she was really seeing.

We paged through the rest of *Femalia*. Even though I had gone through it countless times I was moved, as I often am, by the beauty and diversity of women's vulvas. For Mary Ann it was the first time she'd seen a nonclinical, real-life representation of female genitalia and it was as eye-opening for her as it is for most of us. I hoped she was beginning to question the standard of perfection that she had fixed in her mind and that the range of normal was widening for her.

As we looked at the last of the women profiled in *Femalia*, I asked Mary Ann if she wanted to take a second look at any of the photos. She asked to go back to the woman whose labia hung unevenly.

"I just can't believe it. I wonder if mine is this uneven," she said.

"We can find out," I said.

I explained the mirror exercise. In this case, I suggested we both participate, and that each of us closely examine each body part, from head to toe, and share our thoughts and feelings. I would go first and then it would be Mary Ann's turn.

This exercise is valuable for a number of reasons. It offers clients an opportunity to really examine and think about their bodies. For some, it marks the first time they have ever carefully looked at their whole body. So many of our ideas about our bodies come from unreliable sources. If we've been told that certain areas are bad or ugly or too big or too small, we can believe that without ever really looking to see if the physical reality aligns with our opinion. This exercise offers clients a chance to start formulating their own understanding of their bodies and to compare their beliefs to what they see in front of them. Each client gets something different from this exercise. I thought it would be particularly important for Mary Ann to try to take a dispassionate look at her body, especially after viewing the eye-opening photographs in *Femalia*.

I also hoped that seeing me and carefully looking at herself would help her to shake loose her rigid beliefs about physical perfection. Still, I made it clear that there was no pressure to feel a certain way about any areas of her body. Our goal here was to take an honest inventory, and there were no right or wrong observations.

Together we headed to the bedroom.

We got undressed and I guided Mary Ann through some relaxation exercises.

Then it was time for us to take a tour of our bodies.

⁂

I stood in front of the full-length mirror mounted on my closet door and asked Mary Ann if she was ready to start. I noticed that my legs were a little hairy and my breasts were swollen because I was in the third week of my cycle.

Mary Ann sat up in bed with her legs crossed.

"I haven't seen a naked woman since I was in my high school locker room," she said.

"We don't see a lot of real-life nudity in this culture. It's one reason we have such skewed ideas about what we're supposed to look like," I said.

Mary Ann smiled at my reflection in the mirror and I smiled back at her. I noticed the comma-shaped lines that formed around my mouth as I did.

"So, I'm going to start the exercise. As we discussed, I'll begin at the top and work my way down," I said.

I ran my fingers through my hair, which hung to just below my shoulders.

"I like my hair now. I didn't when I was younger because my mother always told me it was too fine. It feels soft and I like the way it frames my face."

I talked about my face. "I felt self-conscious about my forehead for a long time, again because of my mother. She always told me that it was too big and when I was young she cut my hair in bangs. As I got older I grew more comfortable with it and today I like my face, including my forehead. My skin shows a few more freckles as it's aged, but all in all I like my complexion."

Mary Ann squinted her eyes as if she were trying to get a better look.

"My neck is starting to sag a little, and I'm concerned about getting a waddle under my chin. I like that it is long and it looks pretty when I wear a V-neck shirt with a necklace."

I stretched out my arms.

"I like my shoulders and arms more now that I have built up some muscle in them. I used to think my upper arms were too chubby."

Mary Ann crossed her arms over her chest and squeezed her shoulders.

"My chest is okay. I don't think about it much. I love my breasts." For a moment I paused and thought about how Mary Ann's breasts seemed so out of proportion with her body. The point here, however, was not to try to make the client feel anything—positive or negative. It's simply an inventory, and so I forged on. "I think they are just the right size. The pink of the nipples reminds me of an inner part of a seashell. They were never perky and that used to bother me, but it doesn't anymore."

Next I moved on to my torso. "I don't like that I am high-waisted. Ideally, I would like my stomach to be a little flatter, but it doesn't really bother me that much.

"I think my vulva is beautiful, but I didn't always—especially before I really looked at it. I love the plumpness of my labia. My lovers have told me that I have a pretty vulva and I believe them. It feels good to hear that. When I was growing up I thought my genitals were gross, partly because of how they smelled. I didn't know how to clean under my clitoral hood and I didn't know that women can get smegma, which is just a mixture of sweat and dead skin cells. It can be easily cleaned away. I had no idea about any of that back then. I just thought my genitals were disgusting."

Mary Ann looked down between her legs, then at the reflection of my mons in the mirror.

"I like that my shoulders and hips are an equal width. I think it gives me a solid look. For a long time I thought my hips and butt were too wide. I wished I had fewer curves, but now I love the shape they give me."

I suspected that Mary Ann thought I would be more critical of my body, and I hoped I was providing a contagious model of self-love, even though that wasn't the main purpose of the exercise. With Mary Ann, as with all clients, my goal here is to model an honest appraisal of a body and to examine the many factors that contribute to our body image. Still, I had come to a point where I was at ease with my body, and I thought it would be nice if some of that rubbed off on the hypercritical Mary Ann. I was trying to integrate permission, that is, to let Mary Ann know that it was permissible to like and respect a body that is flawed.

"My legs are long and muscular and they have a nice shape. I like that my thighs are strong, but I don't like how chubby my inner thighs are. I wish my calves were larger. They seem out of proportion with my thighs. My ankles are narrow and I think that's nice. I like the way they look when I'm wearing a skirt and high heels. I like the shape of my feet and how my toes are slightly bowed. Overall, I think I have an attractive, strong body and I am proud of it. If I were to change anything, I would lose a few pounds, but that may not happen because I hate to diet and I love to eat."

Mary Ann and I smiled at each other. I sat on the bed next to her.

"Ready to try it?" I asked.

She nodded, got up from the bed, and stood in front of the mirror.

"Okay. When you're ready, start with your hair and move your way down," I said.

She took her long, black hair in her hands and said, "I am glad that I have naturally black, shiny hair. My husband likes it and so do I."

She traced around her face with her fingertips.

"I think I have a great face now. I had my nose done, so it is smaller and I like that. I've been told in the past that I have nice, high cheekbones."

Her nose looked like a perfectly inverted seven, a shape so artificial that it made me once again wonder about how the notion of perfect has become so divorced from reality.

"My neck still looks young. I wish it were a little longer. I have pretty arms and I like my skin tone over my chest."

At this point Mary Ann crossed her right arm over her chest and took her left breast in her hand.

"My breasts are beautiful now that I've had implants. They used to be too small. When I was a kid I was worried that I would be flat-chested like my mother."

I wondered what Mary Ann's original bosom looked like and how she determined it was too small. In my view, it was now too big and out of proportion with the rest of her beautiful body.

"My stomach is nice and flat and I love my small waist."

Then she placed her right hand over her pubic mound and then the left on top of it.

"From this angle, my vulva looks okay. I'm worried about looking at it more closely, though, because I can feel the difference in my lips and I worry that it is going to be too ugly to look at."

I suggested she take a deep breath and release it slowly. She closed her eyes. When she was finished, I asked if she was ready to continue and she opened her eyes and stared at herself in the mirror again.

"My hips are in a good proportion to my waist because I exercise so much. I wish my butt was a little bigger. My husband once said he wished I had more to grab onto back there. I've thought about having surgery on it. When I was a kid my legs were long and skinny. They looked like stilts and I wished they were shorter. Now, I think they look like a dancer's legs. I've toned them a lot and I love the way they look in tight pants. My ankles and feet are narrow and I like that." She looked at me to indicate that she was finished. The look on her face was neutral, and I felt that she was honest in her appraisal of her body.

"You did a great job, Mary Ann. I learned a lot about how you feel about your body. Was this helpful for you?"

"Well, it made me realize how much of my body I actually like," she said.

We chatted a little more and then she put on her tights, skirt, and blouse and I got into my jeans and T-shirt.

"Next time we'll introduce our vulvas to each other," I said, and then explained the Sexological to her. This exercise would be different for Mary Ann than it was with my male clients. I wouldn't invite her to explore my genitals, for one, and instead of me touching her genitals, I would guide her in an exploration of her own vulva.

When Mary Ann arrived for her second visit, she had her hair pulled back into a French twist and she wore a tight grey sweater. She looked as gorgeous as she had in our first session. I hoped that today, when she finally looked at her vulva closely for the first time, she would see that it was as beautiful as the rest of her.

We talked for a while about how she had been since our first session and she said she had thought often about the images she had seen in *Femalia*. I asked her to share some of her thoughts and she said she was still shocked about how different each woman was and she wondered how it was that she had reached nearly forty without knowing this.

"It's not uncommon. The images we're used to seeing are unrealistic ones. Most people, no matter their age, are stunned by those photos."

I asked Mary Ann if she was ready to do the Sexological. She stood up and I led the way down the hall to the bedroom.

We ran through a series of relaxation exercises. We got undressed and I got the hand mirror and pillows from the closet. We crossed our legs over each other's and I led Mary Ann on a tour of my vulva. I pulled back my clitoral hood and ran my finger around my clitoris. "This is where the smegma we discussed in our last session lives. You can clean it easily by gently retracting your clitoral hood when you're in the shower and putting a little soap and water around it. But keep soap out of your vagina. It's self-cleaning and you don't want to throw off the acid and alkaline balance. It was really a big deal for me to learn about it, even though it seems so simple. It helped me to understand that my genitals weren't inherently bad or disgusting. I could clean them like any other part of my body and remove the odor they gave off."

I invited Mary Ann to give me feedback. She said that she thought my genitals looked tiny compared to hers.

"We have different shapes and they're both perfectly natural. I would even call them beautiful," I said.

When it was her turn, we switched the position of our legs so that Mary Ann's rested on mine. I held the mirror in front of her vulva so she could get a close look.

"What do you think when you look at your genitals this closely?" I asked.

"The left is a little longer, but it's not as uneven as the one picture we saw."

"Can I guide you in some exploration of your vulva?"

"Okay," Mary Ann said shyly.

I asked her to hold back her outer labia with one hand so that the other hand was free.

"With your index finger, circle lightly around your vulva," I said. "Does one side feel more sensitive than the other?" I asked.

"The left."

"Interesting. It's not at all uncommon for women—or men—to feel more reactive on one side of their genitals than the other. It's very natural. Maybe there is a connection with the left side being longer, and maybe not.

"You know, I would guess that other women in your family have similar-shaped labia," I added.

"So, you think it's a family thing?"

"It could be."

Slowly, Mary Ann seemed to be normalizing her labia, getting more comfortable with the idea that an uneven length didn't mean that there was anything wrong.

I asked her to insert her index finger up to her first knuckle into her vagina and explore her G-spot.

"I worry that I might not have one," Mary Ann said.

"Not every woman is extremely sensitive in that area. It's talked about so much that it easy to believe that all women are, but if you're not that's perfectly natural. It doesn't mean that anything is broken or wrong. Just as genitals can look different, they can respond differently as well, despite what you're led to believe."

Mary Anne inserted her finger into her vagina.

"Okay, now hook your finger up toward your pubic bone. Gently feel around and see if there's any spot that feels more pleasurable than another. If there isn't, don't worry. There's nothing wrong. Again, not all women have G-spot sensitivity."

Mary Ann explored and then said, "I guess I'm one of the women who isn't sensitive here."

"And that's alright."

As we untangled our legs Mary Anne said, "I wonder if my husband ever noticed that my lips are slightly uneven."

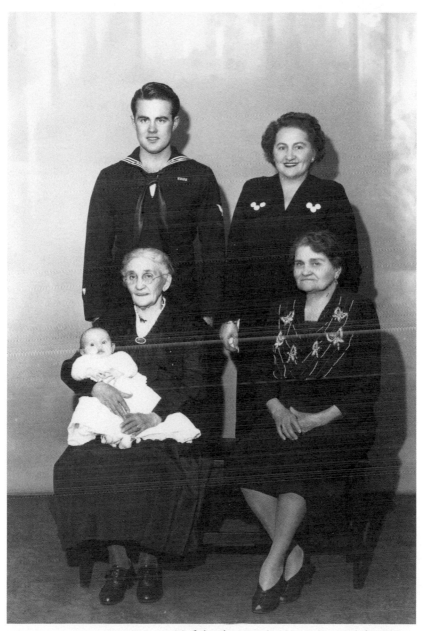

FIVE GENERATIONS. CLOCKWISE: My father, his mom (my Nanna Fournier), her Mom, (my Great Grandmother) and her Mom, (my Great, Great Grandmother) holding me in late 1944.

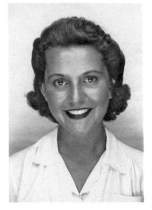

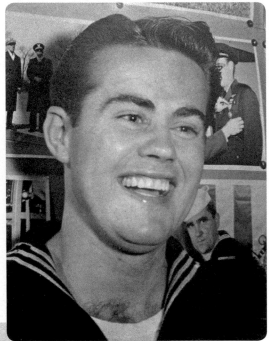

My Mother at 19 in
December 1943.

My Dad at 22 in 1943.

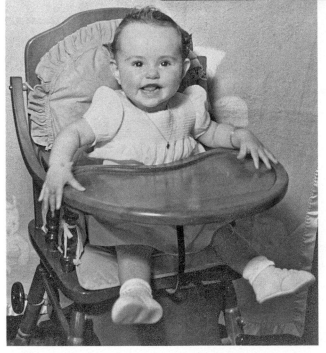

Me at 8 months in
1945.

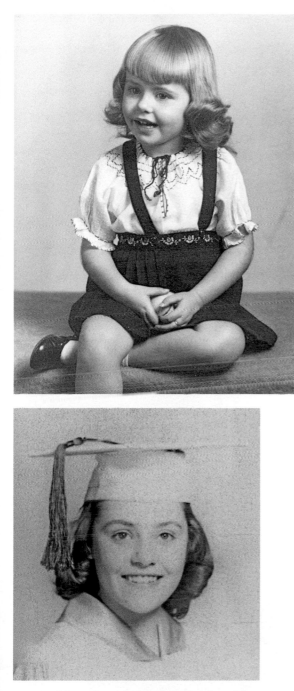

LEFT: Me at 3 in 1947.

BELOW: Me at 12 and my brothers, Peter at 2 and David at 10.

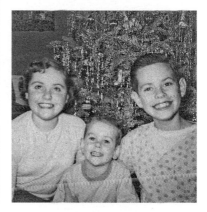

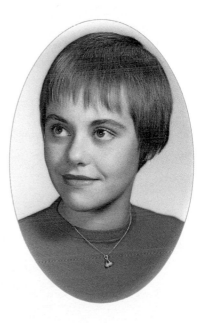

ABOVE: Me at 13, graduating from St. Marys, The Immaculate Conception.

RIGHT: Me at 17, senior yearbook photo from Salem High School.

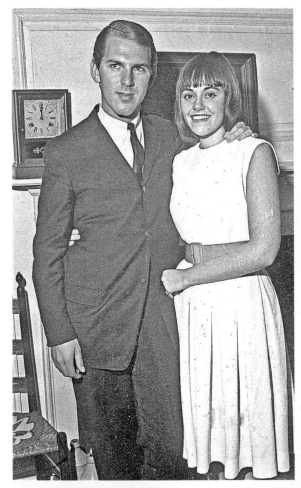

LEFT: Michael and I in early 1964.

BELOW: August 22, 1964. My Mother and me on my wedding day.

BOTTOM: Jessica and me, Summer of 1969.

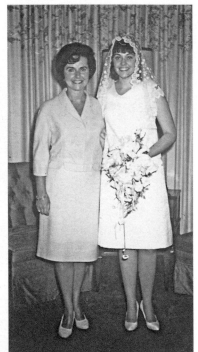

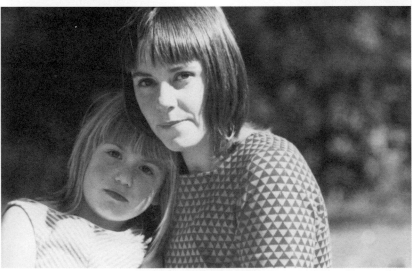

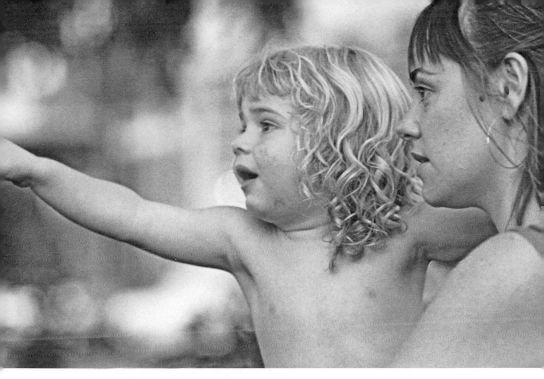

ABOVE: Eric and me, May 1970

LEFT: Michael, Eric, Jessica and me in Summer of 1971.

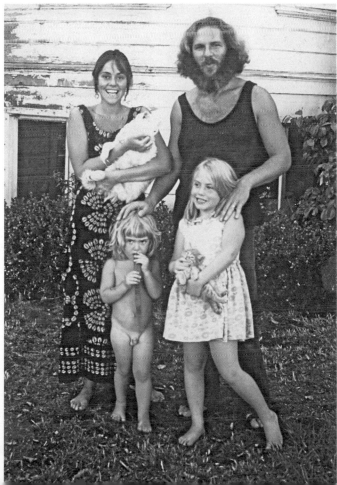

Me in 1973, the year I started Surrogate Partner work.

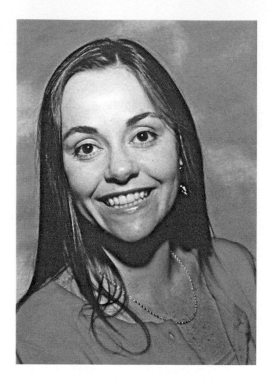

Bob at the University of California Botanical Garden on our first date in 1979.

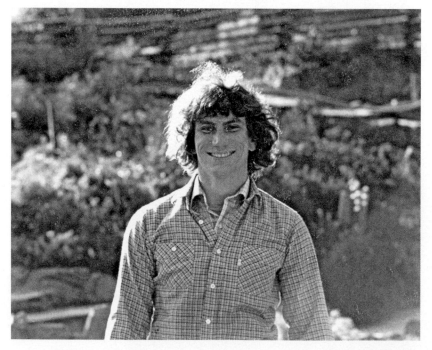

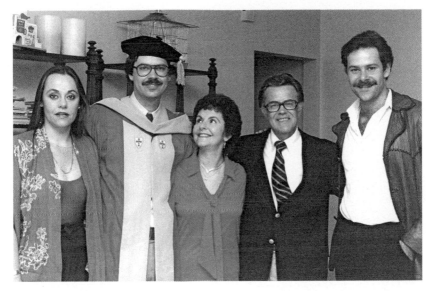

My brother David's graduation from dental school in 1980, with my parents and brother Peter.

Bob and me on our first anniversary in October 1982.

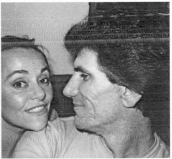

My mother and I in 1983.

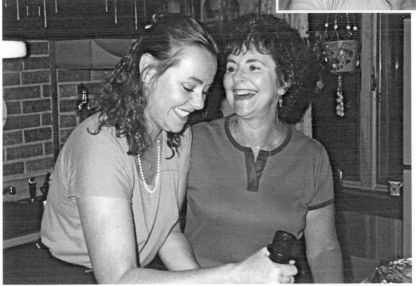

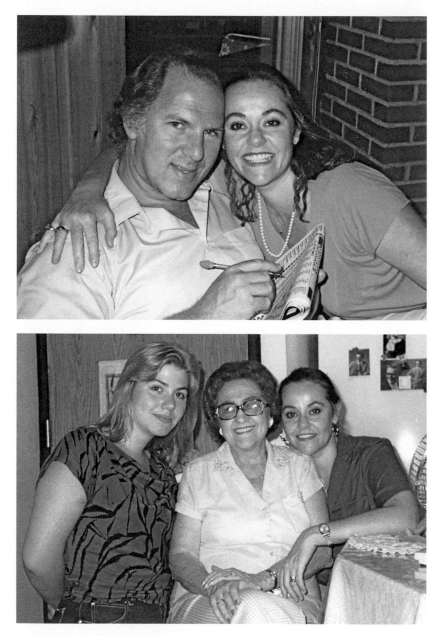

TOP: Michael and me in 1983.   BOTTOM: Jessica, Nanna Fournier and me in Summer of 1984.

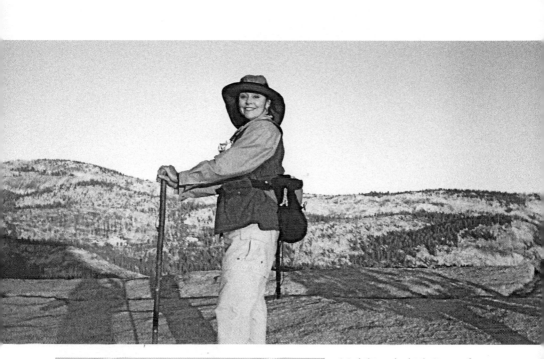

Me hiking the high Sierra of
Yosemite National Park in
September of 1992.

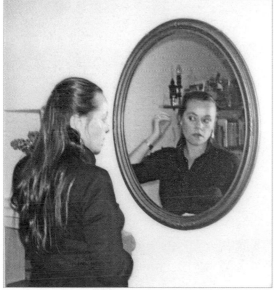

Me in early 1993.

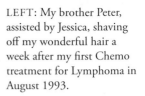

LEFT: My brother Peter, assisted by Jessica, shaving off my wonderful hair a week after my first Chemo treatment for Lymphoma in August 1993.

BELOW: Me midway through my six Chemo treatments. Not quite sure how it would all turn out.

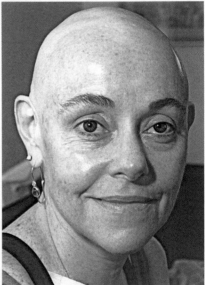

Me feeling a bit more optimistic.

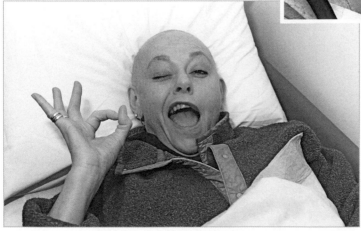

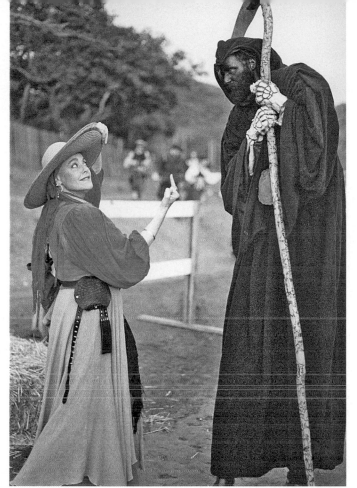

Me giving the finger to the Grim Reaper at the 1993 Renaissance Faire in Novato, CA. after my second chemo treatment.

My chemo was over. I celebrated with my favorite crustacean.

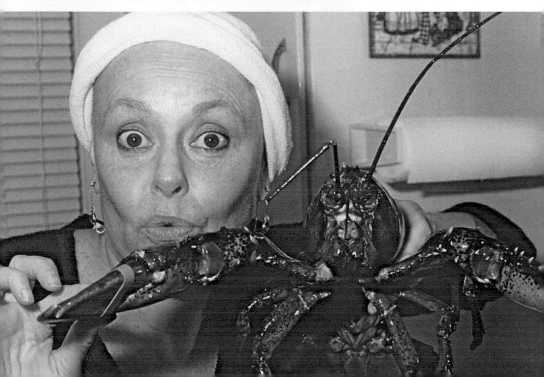

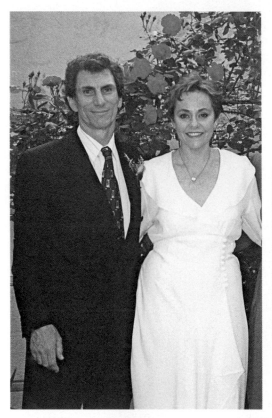

Bob and I were married again. This time for real. April 22, 1995.

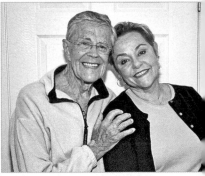

ABOVE: My Dad, at age 88, and me in June 2009.

BELOW: My brothers David (LEFT), Peter and me in October 2010.

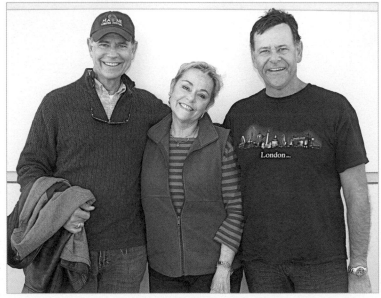

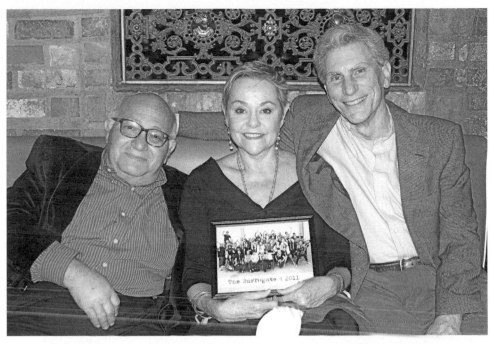

Ben Lewin, Bob and me at the 'Wrap Party' for 'The Surrogate' (later named 'The Sessions'). June 8, 2011.

Helen Hunt and me on June 8, 2011.

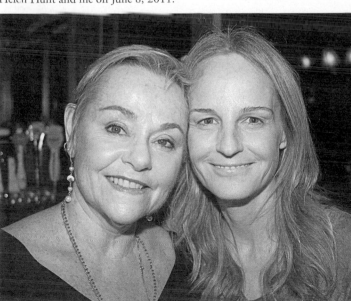

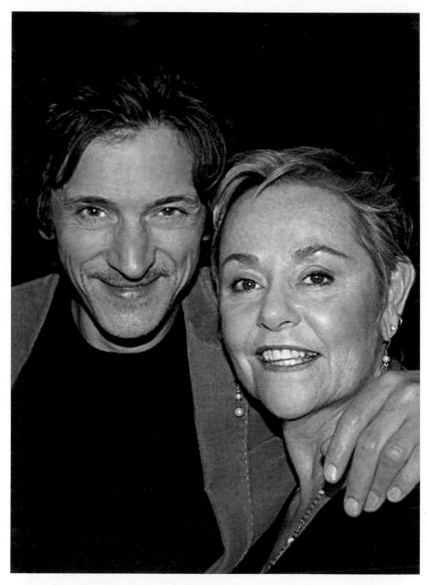

ABOVE: John Hawkes and me on June 8, 2011.

OPPOSITE TOP: My Cousin Susan and me before the party following the premiere of "The Surrogate" on January 23, 2012 at the Sundance Film Festival in Utah.

OPPOSITE BOTTOM: Bob and I at our annual family Oyster Fest at Tomales Bay, October 2011.

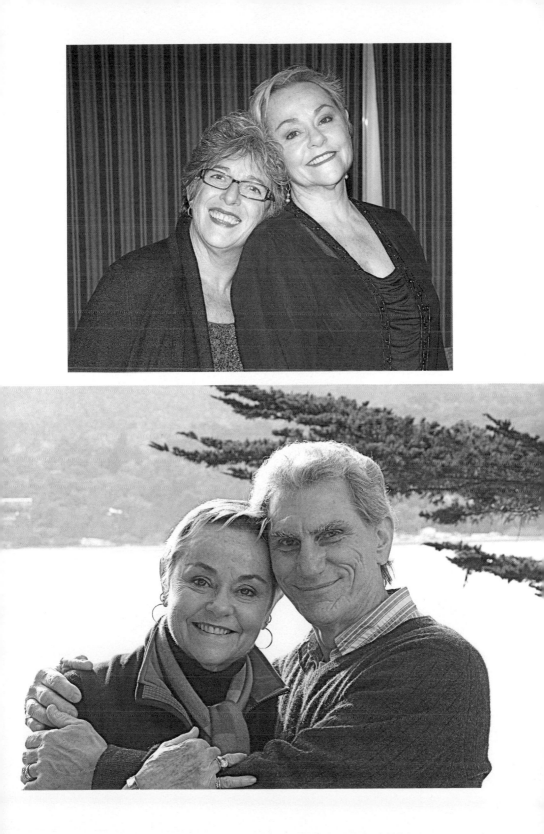

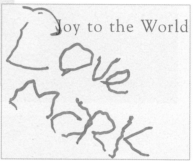

5-29-86

CHERYL,

THANK YOU FOR

all you've

done FOR Me.

MARK

LEFT: Mark O'Brien wrote me this card after our last session.

BELOW: Mark O'Brien sent me this Christmas card in 1998. He died on July 4, 1999 from post-polio syndrome.

Joy to the World

Love MARK

My friend and confidant for nearly half a century, Marshasue Cohen in 2004.

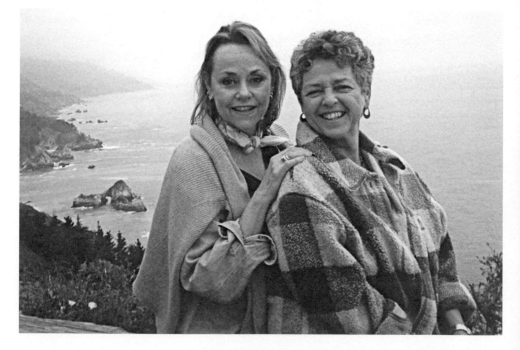

"Is this something you feel you can talk about with him?" I asked.

"I think so now. Before, I just assumed that he noticed and didn't want to hurt my feelings."

Mary Ann's perspective had shifted a little. I believed that the two exercises I had done with her were likely to be effective.

As we parted that day, I told Mary Anne that if she felt she ever wanted to see me again or if she had more questions that she should call me. I called Jodie that night to update her on our last session.

Several months later, Jodie called about another client. She let me know that she was still seeing Mary Ann and that it would take some time to fully address her body image issues, but she no longer believed that her vulva was the problem.

10.

becoming a surrogate

Michael and I hadn't had sex for almost a week. For some couples this would be unremarkable; for us it was a red flag. We had been in California for about a year and suddenly our sex life had dropped off a cliff. When I tried to kiss or cuddle up with him in bed he told me he was sleepy and rolled over onto his side with his back facing me. Michael being too tired for sex was like a fish being too tired to swim. I remembered when he would work a ten-hour shift at his hospital job and then come home and spend hours making love with me. The first couple of nights I tried to convince myself that maybe he was tired. Maybe he just needed some downtime. But when I was rebuffed for the fifth night in a row, I knew something other than fatigue was at play.

On the evening of my sixth day of involuntary abstinence I went to a yoga class; at the end, as I lay in corpse pose with my feet flopped out, palms turned up, and my back pressed against a rubber mat, I started to cry. Anxiety ran through me like a current that couldn't be shut off. Six days without sex was surely a sign of trouble. Was it the first stage of total disengagement? Was this Michael's way of easing out of the relationship?

"Deep breaths. Don't forget to breathe," the willowy yoga teacher said as she walked between the rows of prone students.

I couldn't breathe because my nose was too stuffed up from crying. I sat up, walked over to the doorway of the room where our shoes were lined up against the wall, slipped my feet into mine, and left the class. As I drove home, I decided to talk with Michael. I needed to know what was going on. Even if my worst fear was true, at least I would know what I was dealing with and I could put an end to the speculation that was making me too anxious to relax even in corpse pose.

When I got home, Michael had just put the kids to bed and he stood at the kitchen sink washing dishes. I walked up behind him and put my arms around his waist. He turned on the water to rinse the suds off his hands and then twisted his body around, loosening my embrace. He took a few steps away from the sink with his hands up and grabbed a dishtowel.

"Michael, we need to talk," I said.

"Okay," he answered, and sat down at the kitchen table.

I sat down across from him.

"What's going on? Why aren't we having sex?"

Michael explained that he was feeling performance pressure because I regularly initiated sex.

"When I want sex I'll initiate it," he said.

This rocked me. First, I was humiliated. Was he saying that he didn't want to have sex with me? Was this Michael's way of accusing me of being a sex maniac, à la John, my teenage boyfriend? Also, I thought we were casting off tradition here. Was it suddenly wrong for me to want and initiate sex? I tried hard to maintain my composure, but soon I was crying again.

"Remember back in Boston when I told you that I had never been monogamous?"

I sure did. Michael told me this the first time we slept together. I wanted to think the sheer force of my love would turn him into a one-woman man.

"Well, I don't want to be monogamous now. I need more stimulation," he said.

More stimulation? I felt like the wind had just been knocked out of me. Then he pointed to an issue of the *Berkeley Barb* that lay on top of a pile of papers on our table. "Have you seen the ads for swingers parties in here?"

It took me no time at all to realize that Michael was asking for an open marriage. My feelings were not just mixed, but at odds. In 1970, traditional marriage was one of the many institutions up for popular review. In truth, I was curious about exploring with other men. I was only twenty-five. I had finally shaken off my religious guilt and shame and I was living in the heart of the sexual revolution, the San Francisco Bay Area. Part of me was happy to dispense with the confines of marriage, but another part of me was terrified of losing Michael. But then if I refused, would I push him out of my life completely? I did a quick, barely perceptible calculation and realized that opening the marriage would probably offer me the best chance at keeping it.

That night as I lay beside Michael, watching his chest rise and fall to the rhythm of his even breathing, I thought about our life together, about what I wanted it to be, and about what it was in reality. I remembered one evening back in Boston when Michael, his friend Ron, and I spent most of the night talking in my apartment. Somehow we got on the subject of cheating. Michael asserted that if he was attracted to a friend's girlfriend, he saw nothing wrong with sleeping with her behind his friend's back. Ron fired back that that was a betrayal of the friendship, but Michael held his ground. If both people were interested, why should they deny themselves? There was plenty of reason to know that no matter how much I loved him or how special I imagined our relationship to be, Michael would never limit himself to me.

On a brisk Saturday night a couple of weeks later, we left the kids with some friends and headed to Concord, a bedroom community about fifteen miles east of Berkeley, for our first swingers party. Michael, who rarely wore anything other than jeans and a T-shirt, donned a pair of dress pants and a button-down twill shirt. He even had combed back his hair. I remember thinking that my husband looked like he was going on a first date with a woman he wanted to impress.

It was easy to recognize the house where the party was being held because the driveway and the street in front of it were clogged with sedans. Michael maneuvered the yellow submarine behind a mammoth Lincoln and a red Chevy Impala. I wanted to grab his arm as we walked up to the front door, but instead I kept both my hands wedged into the pockets of my skirt.

Michael smoothed out his shirt before he rang the doorbell. Through the frosted glass of the door window the group of people standing in the foyer looked ghostly. I was trying to make out the ratio of men to women when our host opened the door. Her hair was styled in a beehive and lacquered into place. She wore a blue polyester jumper over a white blouse that tied into a huge bow at her neck. I could detect a change in her skin tone along her jaw where her heavy pancake makeup ended. She took our coats and my purse and led us into the sunken living room. I quickly scanned the crowd, which I judged almost immediately as decidedly unhip. If Michael expected a grotto of lolling bohemian beauties he had wildly miscalculated and I was tickled because of it.

I turned to say something to Michael and discovered he was already mingling. As I made my way through the crowd, several men, none of whom I found attractive, ogled me. I felt like I was being looked at like a new piece of meat. We were supposed to be scaling the heights of sexual adventurism and all I could think was, Is this how a new prison inmate feels?

I poured a glass of wine and pretended to examine our hosts' record collection. As I flipped through the rows of LPs in the cabinet next to the stereo, a few intrepid men approached me, but I was about as welcoming as a dentist's drill.

Many of the guests had paired off and were having sex on the shag-carpeted living room floor. As I pretended to read the back cover of a Neil Diamond record, I noticed Michael out of the corner of my eye chatting with the one woman in the crowd who was his type. She was tall and slender and her dark hair hung down just below her chin. She had a pointy nose and chiseled cheekbones.

"Having fun?"

I looked away from Michael and found our host standing next to me.

"Oh yes. It's great. Thanks for having us."

"Looks like your husband's met Nina. Did you know she just made her debut at the San Francisco Opera?"

"No, I didn't. Isn't that wonderful."

"Yup, she's got a gorgeous voice—a soprano."

"Fantastic."

I drained my glass.

"Time for a refill," I said and walked across the room to the bar.

So, Michael was chatting up a diva. At that point I had some very particular ideas about how to raise his voice a few octaves.

I sat down on the couch and nursed my wine. I watched as the conversation between Michael and Nina heated up. He touched her arm. She smiled and ruffled his hair. They kissed. Before long they were one of the writhing couples on the floor. I told myself to stop watching, but I could barely blink. What really upset me was that Michael was doing stuff with her that he did with me. He was going down on her and she was wriggling with delight. I wanted to believe this was reserved for me, his wife, the one who was special enough to marry. Neither one noticed me staring at them. About four other couples were splayed out on the spacious floor, and at least two of them were having intercourse. People buzzed around as if it were normal to have to step over copulating couples to get to the other side of the living room. It was all so tawdry.

Finally, I pulled myself off the couch and went out onto the deck. I leaned against the redwood railing, the cool night air pressed against my burning face. I looked up at the moon and out over the hills. It was a big world filled with lots of people. Seeing Michael with someone else hurt, but I reminded myself that I, too, now had the freedom to wander.

I left the party without even speaking to another man, and I was pretty quiet on the drive back home. I knew the boundaries and rules I had been raised with would have never worked for me. They would have led to a life of misery. But should there be no boundaries? Was Michael's contrarianism really just a guise for his hedonism, a convenient vehicle for selfish behavior? Once again I felt myself pulled in opposite directions. I was hurt. I didn't want to share Michael, but at the same time I was curious. I wanted to redraw the boundaries. At this point, I just had no idea where.

⟡

I had always wanted four children, but with our tenuous financial circumstances Michael and I decided to stop at two. For now, we would concentrate on raising our two wonderful children with as much love and attention as we could possibly give them. Also, an open marriage was complicated enough. The last thing I wanted was to get pregnant by another man.

I tried taking the Pill, but it caused my mood to do gymnastics. One minute I was cheerful and content, the next I was crying and battling despair. So I opted instead for an IUD, called a Lippes Loop. It was painless and I didn't have to remember to take a pill every day or endure mood swings the size of the Grand Canyon.

One day, about three months after the Lippes Loop had been implanted, I was in the shower and I noticed that the strings attached to it pushed out farther than normal. I pushed my finger up and felt something protruding out from my cervix. It was blunt at the end and about as wide as a toothpick. My IUD had come loose. I tugged on the strings and eased the Lippes Loop out of my cervix. As it exited, it sprung back into a double-S shape. I stepped out of the tub, toweled off, and called my doctor.

A few days later I sat in his office wrapped in a paper gown.

"Yes, Miss . . . Mrs. Cohen," Dr. Sutton said as he looked down at my chart.

"Well, as I mentioned to the nurse my IUD—"

"Yes, I heard all about it. What is it you'd like me to do?"

"I was wondering about getting it replaced."

"Really? Well, I can't promise that it won't come out, and since you're afraid of the Pill, maybe we should try another alternative that will save us both some time."

He opened a drawer and took out something that looked like a guitar pick with legs.

"This," he pumped his hand, "is the Dalkon Shield, and it won't come out."

It was possible that Dr. Sutton just had an awful bedside manner, or that he didn't respect women in general, or that he was too arrogant to show any sensitivity to any of his patients. Sure, it was possible, but what I believed then and still do today is that he had contempt for me because I was on welfare. I suspected that his well-heeled patients saw a whole other side of him.

"I—okay—I guess so," I said.

Dr. Sutton told me to get up on the table and put my feet in the stirrups. He opened my vagina with a speculum and pushed the Dalkon Shield into my uterus. The pain took my breath away. He peeled off his latex gloves and said, "You can get dressed now," and left the room.

The new IUD remained uncomfortable. At first I thought that maybe it was because it was new, but a week later, and then two weeks later, it still felt painful. Unlike the Lippes Loop, I could never forget the Dalkon Shield was jammed into my uterus. After about a month I made another appointment with Dr. Sutton, whose only response was, "Well, that's what you wanted to use, wasn't it? You don't want to use the Pill." I was too intimidated to question him, even though I knew something was wrong.

The new IUD also made sex less pleasurable, both with Michael and my new lover, Jeff, who I had met through a friend. Jeff was smart, artistic, and adventurous. He wasn't conventionally handsome, but his personality was so vital that it hardly mattered. He had a sleek new red Mustang and we often drove up to Marin County or down to Santa Cruz and found a secluded place to make love.

About three months after I began using the Dalkon Shield, Jeff picked me up one Sunday evening and we hit the Great Highway, landing at the beach. I had been feeling a deep ache in my lower abdomen for a few days that was unlike the discomfort I normally felt from my new IUD. I hoped it would go away and I didn't take it terribly seriously, in part because I'd grown accustomed to ignoring the pain. I reclined back in the passenger seat, put my feet up on the dashboard, and held Jeff's hand. We looked out over the ocean and watched the sun sink into it. We kissed for a few minutes. Then I pulled away and told Jeff I needed to pee. I walked to the front of the car and squatted down so that the few other people in the parking lot couldn't see me. A few drops trickled out, burning as they escaped. I looked down at a quarter-size circle of urine on the ground below me. Suddenly, I was seized with the most excruciating pain I had ever felt. It was worse than childbirth, worse than the pain after the car wreck. I felt like the inside of my vagina was being invaded by a knife. The pain was so bad I couldn't stand up. I passed out for a few seconds and when I came to I managed to clutch the bumper of the car and straighten out my legs enough to limp to the driver's side.

"Get me home. Please. Something's terribly wrong," I panted.

"Oh Christ, what's going on?" Jeff cried.

"Get me home. Get me home," I pleaded.

He lay me down in the backseat of the Mustang and got onto the road. I passed out again. Jeff shook my arm and when I came to I saw his head snap forward to look back at the road.

The next time I woke up, Michael was carrying me out of Jeff's car and into his, where I drifted away again and didn't wake up until I was in the emergency room. Michael and a nurse poured me into a wheelchair. I was taken straight to an exam room, where the last person in the world I wanted to see soon walked in. Dr. Sutton happened to be on duty that night. By now, the pain was so great that it hurt to breathe.

"Lie back and spread your legs. I need to examine you," Dr. Sutton said.

He took some swabs of my vagina, inserted his fingers, and felt around. I was in excruciating pain throughout his brutal examination. All the while he was talking to the nurse who stood beside him.

"Get those to the lab and call Dr. Ivy," he said, still inside of me.

Then, without saying a word to me, he ripped out the Dalkon Shield. I screamed so loudly that Michael came running into the room. I wasn't sure how much more pain I could endure.

I was admitted to the hospital and the next morning I learned that I had infectious peritonitis, cervicitis (inflammation of the cervix), and pelvic inflammatory disease. In short, I was a mess. Later tests showed that my fallopian tubes were so scarred that it was highly unlikely that I would ever get pregnant again. As it turned out, this wasn't an uncommon outcome for many of the hundreds of thousands of women who used the now notorious Dalkon Shield. At twenty-six I was done having children. Even though Michael and I agreed to have only two, in the back of my mind I always thought I had time to reconsider.

I had been in California for two years, and in that time I had survived a major car accident and now this ordeal. I was beginning to wonder if anything good would happen to me again. Maybe I should have just stayed in Boston. Compared to what I was going through now, my parents, the New England winters, and all of the other things I had complained about didn't seem so bad.

In reality, there was no going back, and it hadn't been all gloom and doom. I'd made some wonderful friends in California. They were young people who had come from all over the country, people like me who were questioning what they had been taught and who were experimenting with alternative lifestyles and new ways of thinking.

As the years passed, I became confident that I had made the right decision. Sure, we had had a rocky start, but moving to California afforded me all sorts of opportunities and experiences that I never would have had back in Massachusetts. In 1973, five years after my move across country, my friend Alison invited me to an event that reminded me how far I was from Salem and started me on a career path I would never have dreamed of in my earlier life.

Alison asked me to attend a talk on sex at a church (a church!) in Berkeley. It was being led by three women who had just founded San Francisco Sex Information (SFSI, pronounced Sfissy), one of the first telephone hotlines for unbiased, fact-based sex education in the country. "Sexual ignorance is not bliss" is SFSI's motto.

Alison and I had dinner at a small café a few blocks away from the church. As we often did, we got lost in conversation and didn't leave until about ten minutes to seven. Neither of us was worried, though. We had only a short way to walk. As we reached the church we saw a line that snaked around the building. Would we get in? Alison and I took our places in line, shocked at the turnout. As it started to move we grew less optimistic that we would make it in. The church was obviously too small to hold everyone who wanted to attend. As I got near the doorway, I looked in and saw a sea of people, many of them standing. Alison walked in and I followed. Just as I stepped inside I heard the greeter apologize to the people behind me who had to be turned away because there was simply no more room left.

The evening started with a film that I will never forget. It followed a woman as she masturbated and reached climax. This wasn't only shocking because of what she was doing, but because of who she was. This was a normal-looking woman, with an imperfect body that she seemed perfectly at ease with. The star of the film was Shirley Lewis.

When the movie ended and the lights came on, the stark silence of the room was almost palpable. A few moments later Alison turned to me and asked, "Do you ever do that?" When I nodded my head yes, she replied, in a kind of conspiratorial whisper, "So do I." So, other women liked sex too? We broke up into discussion groups and I found that I was far from alone, not just in my shame, but also in my confusion and anger about how my sexuality had been treated within the Church, my family, and society. This was the first time I had ever been encouraged to talk openly and publicly about masturbation or any other sexual practice. Times were indeed a-changin'.

The next morning when I told Michael about the event, the first of two serendipitous things happened. Turned out, Michael, who had been taking a class at the now-defunct Center for Intimacy, knew Shirley. In fact, she taught the class he was taking. Michael mentioned to Shirley how impressed I was with her and he learned that, in addition to her work as an educator, she was also a surrogate partner. Then, about a week later, my friend Elizabeth gave me a copy of *Surrogate Wife* by Valerie X. Scott, who had been a Masters and Johnson–trained surrogate. The coincidences were starting to mount, and I began to wonder what it might be like to be a surrogate myself.

I wasn't alone anymore. Many people struggled with issues around sexuality and maybe I could help them. I no longer had to apologize for being a woman who enjoyed having sex. I still didn't know if I liked it more or less than other women, but I was starting to think that it didn't matter if I did. It occurred to me that maybe I could even actively channel a strong libido into something that would help individuals feel happier and, I hoped, might make the world a better place.

I contacted Shirley to learn more about what exactly a surrogate did. No, they didn't just show up and have sex with a client. There was a protocol that lasted, on average, six to eight visits. It could be shorter or longer depending on the client's needs, and there were specific exercises designed to address the most common sexual problems. Surrogates worked closely with traditional talk therapists and all of their clients were referred by them. They worked with both couples and individuals. Most of the people they saw struggled with premature ejaculation, delayed ejaculation, erectile dysfunction, lack of desire, little or no sexual experience, poor body image, anxiety, physical disability, or some combination of these issues. A keen sense of compassion and a deep capacity for empathy were essential because, as a surrogate, you helped people address some of the most deeply personal, anxiety-provoking issues that they would ever face. Potential surrogates also must have addressed their own issues with sexuality.

The practice of surrogacy originated with Masters and Johnson, whose groundbreaking research in the 1950s and '60s popularized the study of human sexuality. William Masters and Virginia Johnson were married researchers who did some of the earliest scientific work on the human sexual response and sexual dysfunction. Their books, *Human Sexual Response* and *Human Sexual Inadequacy*, were bestsellers and some of the first works to demystify sexuality. At their center in St. Louis they trained the very first surrogates and created the template for the process we use today.

Originally, Masters and Johnson worked with married couples who were struggling with a variety of sexual issues. Later, they opened their practice to single men and the profession of surrogacy was born. Another pair of married researchers, William E. Hartman and Marilyn Fithian, developed additional exercises and wrote a number of insightful books, including *Treatment of Sexual Dysfunction*. They worked with surrogate partners in California who were trained by Caroline and Emerson Symonds, two highly-respected sexologists. At the Center for Social and Sensory Learning in Southern California, Barbara M. Roberts, MSW, began training surrogates and therapists as well as offering workshops for the public. Shirley referred me to two therapists who worked well with surrogates and in a few days I had an appointment with one of them in Berkeley.

By this time, my marriage had been open for almost five years and I had enjoyed my share of sexual partners. Michael and I had come to a working agreement about how we would handle outside relationships.

We wouldn't let them interfere with our time with our children. We would only go out one night a week each, and one of us would stay home with Jessica and Eric. If one of us came home late, there was no sleeping in the next day. We got up at the same time the next morning to make breakfast and get the kids off to school. When I discussed my new career course with Michael he was supportive and I don't think this was just another example of Michael's disquieting lack of jealousy. I believe he truly understood the value of this work and wanted to see me find a career that I could embrace and nurture. If Michael had ever had conventional attitudes about sex, he had jettisoned them so long ago that it wouldn't occur to him to be critical of this profession. He also understood that traditional mores about sex needed to evolve, and if surrogacy could play a small role in helping with that, so much the better.

Tom greeted me with a welcoming smile. He was one of only a few therapists in the Bay Area (San Francisco) who were training surrogates and referring clients to them. The field was in its infancy and the training was rapidly evolving. We talked for two hours and Tom asked me questions about my background, my relationship with my family, and my attitude toward sex. We had an instant rapport. I think Tom understood immediately that I was well past the point in my own sexual evolution where I would demonize anyone for having a sexual problem. It would be the first step in our training together. Then Tom asked me to do something that made me suspicious. "Why don't you take off your clothes so I can see what you'd look like with clients," he said. Was this his way of hitting on me? Also, I didn't shave my legs or my underarms at the time. I wondered what he would have to say about that. Our meeting had gone well and I liked Tom, so I decided to take a chance. I pulled my loose-fitting dress over my head and took off my underwear. "You look good to me," Tom said. I was relieved that he didn't make a pass at me, but I still thought it was inappropriate. I wanted to be a surrogate, not a fashion model. Did my body really need to be cleared before I could start training? Tom never mentioned another word to me about this, so, if it was a test, I supposed I had passed.

I also began training to be a phone counselor at SFSI. They had established an 800 number for people to call with questions about sex. For one of the first times in U.S. history people could pick up the phone, ask questions anonymously, and get reliable information and referrals for expert help. In my initial interview with a SFSI staffer I was asked a number of questions and several hypothetical scenarios were put to me. For example, my interviewer asked what I would do when callers said that they feared they were masturbating too much. "I would ask them what they meant by 'too much.' If they're masturbating because they are afraid to meet someone or if it's getting in the way of normal daily functioning, like going to work, I'd refer them to a therapist. If they're doing it because it's pleasurable and relieves stress, I'd probably tell them that it's perfectly natural," I answered.

SFSI training allowed me to be an effective phone volunteer, and it also augmented my surrogacy education. As part of the training, we watched films of people engaging in a variety of sexual practices and then discussed our reactions to them. We were encouraged to talk frankly and to honestly examine our responses and what they might tell us about ourselves. The movies showed heterosexual sex and both male and female homosexual sex. One showed an older couple—and I mean as old as my grandparents—making passionate love. To my surprise, I got aroused when I watched a film of gay men having sex. When I saw one of a man and woman having anal sex I was both excited and repelled. Taboo can be a turn on.

Through discussions with fellow trainees and SFSI staffers I realized that what was more important than my visceral reactions was my ability to suspend my judgment of the consensual acts I had witnessed, and of the people who called for information or help. It was okay if a particular practice didn't appeal to me. What would make me an effective educator and sounding board was not the range of my sexual repertoire, but my ability to empathize and maintain objectivity.

A key part of my surrogacy training came when I attended a two-week workshop with Tom at the Department of Public Health in Berkeley. If Tom had made a misstep in our initial meeting by asking to see my body, he had redeemed himself by being so generous with his time and expertise. The workshop was led by a husband-and-wife therapist team who had trained with Masters and Johnson. They laid out the principles and practice of conjoint therapy. Few professionals use this model today because it is not cost-effective, but at the time it was an exciting new form of couples therapy. It was always conducted by a male-female team, and the hope was that both partners in the couple would feel that they had an ally. In the workshop, we got a crash course in anatomy and for the first time I learned the complexity of both male and female genitalia. They showed us the undifferenti-ated genital chart, which I continue to use in my practice today. It reveals how the fetus differentiates into male or female and the simi-larities in genital tissue. Much of what Tom and I learned became part of my surrogacy work.

Between my training to be a surrogate and my SFSI training, my knowledge of human sexuality exploded. I realized just how many assumptions and misconceptions I harbored. I met people from all walks of sexual life and many of the biases I held about them were challenged. For example, I always thought people who were involved in sadism and masochism (S&M) had to be pretty unsavory. To my surprise, I learned that they took great care not to cause any real harm during sex play. Ironically, another thing I learned was that it was okay to say no. People didn't have to continue with or engage in any activity just because they were taking a more open and experimental attitude toward sex. This may not seem noteworthy now, but for someone who grew up in the '50s it was a real eye-opener to be told that, even as a woman, I had the right to choose or not choose any kind of sex, no matter the circumstances.

One absolutely invaluable skill I learned was how to listen. This was tough because I love to talk! In both my SFSI and surrogate training I had to learn how not to jump in, but rather give people the space they needed to say what they wanted to say. This made me a better surrogate, but it also made me a better wife, mother, and friend.

I became part of a wonderful, intelligent, and supportive community of people who were questioning, sharing, and seeking genuine knowledge about sexuality. I was on my way to a meaningful career, making lasting friendships, and, frankly, having a hell of a lot of fun.

One thing we didn't discuss was safe sex and the use of condoms. Because of my Dalkon Shield nightmare I was at very low risk of getting pregnant. In this pre-AIDS era the greatest fear was herpes. Most other STDs could be cured with a stiff dose of antibiotics. I knew this not just because of all of my recent training, but because five years earlier I had a brush with venereal disease when one week after the swingers party in Concord, we got a call from our host: The diva had gonorrhea.

11.

more than a client: bob

In 1979, the Canon AE-1 was a camera that any serious amateur photographer would have been happy to own. When my client Bob handed it to me, along with its motor-drive accessory, I had to use both hands to hold it. It weighed probably five times as much as my Instamatic, and its lens was ringed with number sequences that looked like some kind of code.

"I can't accept this," I said.

Just a few minutes ago, Bob had sat in the bathroom chatting with me while I took a shower. When I closed my eyes to rinse the shampoo out of my hair the room went quiet. I opened them and he was gone. I stepped out of the shower stall, towel-dried my hair, and wrapped myself in a terrycloth robe. "Bob?" I called. Just as I walked out of the bathroom I saw him coming down the hall toward me with the camera in his hand.

"It's way too generous," I said.

Bob blinked back tears.

"I really want you to have it. You've changed my life, Cheryl, and this is my way of saying thank you. Please, let me do this."

I knew why he had chosen a camera. In one of our early sessions Bob had told me about his love of photography and how he had set up a dark room in his closet at home. I mentioned that I had missed capturing so many precious moments in my children's lives because I didn't have a reliable camera or much skill in using the one I had.

"Bob, this is so sweet, really, but I wouldn't know how to use it."

"I could teach you," he said quietly. "How about I come down here on my day off and show you. It's easy. We can go to the park and take some outdoor shots."

"Hmmm, I guess so. Okay, let's do it." I said.

With that, I made a date with one of my clients. That was the last of our eight sessions together and a personal relationship had tentatively bloomed alongside our professional one for the last few weeks of our work together.

Because of his work Bob was almost always my last client of the day. We started our sessions at around four in the afternoon and he normally stuck around afterward, talking to me while I showered and got made up in my office bathroom before he walked me to my car.

When he first came to see me, Bob was thirty years old, four years my junior. He had a friendly face framed by wavy, shoulder-length hair. He was ruggedly handsome. Perhaps it was the pensiveness in his eyes or the way he hesitated before he crossed my office doorway, but the first thing I thought when I saw him was that he had a gentle soul.

I sensed his nervousness the minute he walked in, so I made small talk. As we chatted, I saw his anxiety abate a little. His shoulders dropped and he let his back, which he had held as straight as a pool cue, relax to the point where he allowed himself to lean back in the overstuffed chair across from me.

During our first session, I'd asked Bob to tell me a little about his sexual history.

The shyness I saw in him had been with him for as long as he could remember. It was one reason why he didn't have a girlfriend in high school. Another was that he had facial scarring caused by acne that made him too self-conscious. At times it seemed like he was the only boy in his high school who was too awkward to reel in a girlfriend. He was quietly attracted to many of the girls at school and more than once he watched wistfully as a friend paired off with one of his secret crushes.

In late 1968, just as he turned twenty, Bob was drafted into the army; after a year of training, he was sent to Vietnam, where he was assigned to the 101st Airborne Division as a parachute rigger. It was October 1970 when he took his R & R in Bangkok, where prostitution was legal and regulated by the government. The short flight to Thailand was full of raucous and horny young soldiers. Bob sat in quiet excitement and thought about how he would soon accomplish something that he felt was long overdue: losing his virginity. He felt a combination of apprehension, anticipation, and giddiness about this impending rite of passage.

When he arrived in Bangkok he checked into a hotel, unpacked, and then headed into the steamy night. He soon found a taxi driver who drove him along the well-traversed route to a local "massage parlor." As he opened the front door of a nondescript building, Bob was led by the Mamasan through a dimly lit hallway that spilled into a large room. There stood a small crowd of other GIs with big grins on their faces gazing through a one-way mirror at several scantily clad women perched on plushly carpeted bleachers. They were casually reading or chatting with one another, each with a number pinned to her blouse. "Fifteen, twelve, eight, seventeen . . . " The soldiers rattled off their choices. It was a scene he could only think of as bizarre and it jolted his middle-class American sensibilities to the core. When it was his turn, Bob quietly selected a lovely, mature-looking woman and paid the Mamasan $25 for twenty-four hours.

He flagged a taxi and went back to the hotel with the woman, whose name was Chamneon (pronounced Chom-Nee-In). Once in his room, she slowly and confidently began to undress herself, while Bob tried to fill the awkward silence with small talk. Bob took off his clothes and they got into bed. Chamneon was exotically beautiful. He had fantasized the whole way back to the hotel about making love to her. They kissed softly and then passionately, their tongues darting around each other's mouths. He cupped her small breasts and ran his hands along her smooth back and stomach until he got to her vulva. He fingered her clitoris and she wrapped her long fingers around his penis, which, to Bob's dismay, seemed like it had gone to sleep. What was going on? he wondered. It wasn't like he couldn't get erections. He masturbated as much as any healthy twenty-year-old male. Why now, with a willing and naked woman next to him, did his penis remain flaccid?

He reached for his Thai-English phrasebook and thumbed through it frantically. He wanted to tell Chamneon that he would just need a minute or two. He said a few garbled Thai words to his perplexed date. In retrospect he saw how comical this must have looked, but at the time he was too embarrassed and confused to find anything funny about it. He lay with his arm around Chamneon. He tried a few more times to get hard, but each attempt ended in frustration.

It turned out that Chamneon spoke a little English. Bob discovered this as they talked for much of the night. He learned that she was a twenty-five-year-old single mother to an eight year-old girl. She had left a physically abusive husband and now supported herself, her daughter, and the rest of her family with the only job available to her. Bob started to feel real warmth and sympathy for Chamneon.

While he was disappointed about not losing his virginity, he tried to keep his perspective. He was, after all, in a foreign country with an unfamiliar culture and language. He was with a prostitute who, most likely, was relieved by his glitch. He would give himself a break for his failure and try again.

The next evening Bob returned to the brothel. He ran into some of the same servicemen he had seen the night before, but unlike them he wasn't there to sample a different woman. He paid to have Chamneon for the rest of the week. He enjoyed her company as she showed him around the enigmatic city.

Chamneon took Bob to The Grand Palace, The Temple of the Reclining Buddha, and the stunning beaches on the Bay of Bangkok, where they walked in the surf. Each night when they returned to his hotel room, he tried unsuccessfully to get an erection and have intercourse. Soon the week was over and he returned to Vietnam still a virgin.

"I often wonder what became of Chamneon," Bob said.

"Did you try again with anyone else before coming home?"

"No, I was too discouraged. I took another R & R in Australia, but stayed away from the prostitutes. I was probably the only one of my friends who did."

Shortly thereafter, with his two-year commitment to Uncle Sam fulfilled, Bob found himself on a chartered jet with 150 other ecstatic GI's heading back to "the world." He had plenty of time for reflection on the fourteen-hour flight.

"I decided to wipe the slate clean, to forget about my experience in Bangkok and to just focus on finding a woman I could love. I thought the sex would naturally follow. I thought I just needed to be in love with a woman for my plumbing to function properly. If I just relaxed, it would happen."

He returned home from Vietnam more mature and with a good measure of confidence. He could handle himself in tough situations and knowing this gave him hope that he would get past his personal troubles. When he looked around, he saw couples everywhere. If they can do it, so can I, he told himself. Also, he was only twenty-three. Maybe some of his friends got started earlier, but he was still young enough for his virginity to be unremarkable.

Bob met Jane at work. She was statuesque with a pretty face framed by long black curly hair. She was quiet yet friendly, and he was attracted to her instantly. After some shy flirting, Bob took a chance and told her he had two tickets to see George Carlin and asked if she wanted to join him. Bob soon realized, much to his surprise and delight, that his strong feelings of affection were reciprocated.

"I was flying high as a kite. I finally knew what all the talk about the thrill of first love was about," he said.

That summer Jane quit her job to work at a tiny resort near Yosemite. She encouraged Bob to visit her as soon as he could. Two weeks later he found himself driving with much anticipation up Route 120 for a long weekend tryst with Jane. He couldn't remember ever having been happier.

He and Jane hiked the enchanting High Sierra backcountry trails together. At night they retreated to his mattress-equipped van, and enjoyed energetic and delicious foreplay. They pleasured each other with their mouths and hands, but when it came time for intercourse Bob suddenly stalled. He felt a familiar sense of dread well up in him. Once again, he couldn't get an erection. Sweet Jane tried to comfort him. She assured him that this was just an anomaly and soon they would have intercourse that was as sublime as their foreplay.

"I wanted to believe her, but this time I was mortified and deeply disappointed with myself. I couldn't blame my surroundings any-more," Bob said.

He tried another few times with Jane, but an unfortunate pattern had been set. The intimacy and excitement would build between them and then he would panic, tense up, and think back to his other false starts. As much as he was attracted to Jane, and as much as he craved sex and intimacy with her, he couldn't get an erection.

"I tried to reassure Jane that it wasn't her, but I think she came to believe that I just wasn't attracted to her." She didn't know how to deal with it. She had never encountered a situation like that before.

After several more long weekend visits to Yosemite, Jane lost interest and started avoiding him. His letters went unanswered.

Bob was crushed, and he sank into a depression that didn't lift for several years. He blamed himself. He was trapped in loneliness and saw no escape. He thought of it as a kind of self-imposed solitary confinement. He was his own jailer, except he didn't have the key for his release.

"Did you see a professional for your depression at that time?" I asked.

"I saw a psychiatrist for a few months, but it didn't help. But at my last appointment he did give me the number for the UC San Francisco Human Sexuality Department. He told me that they could refer me to a therapist who worked with surrogates. That was five years ago. I couldn't call them until now."

"What made you finally do it?"

"I know I have to change. I can't go through life like this anymore. I'm tired of being lonely and I'm tired of hating myself. What have I got to lose at this point?"

Bob had a textbook case of performance anxiety. He was mired in the vicious circle that he recognized in himself, and it was my job to help him break it.

Throughout our work together, I did a number of exercises with him. Sensual Touch was one of the most important because it took his focus away from his penis and broadened it to his whole body. I wanted him to experience sensuality and pleasure and let his penis follow along in any way it wanted. We did the Sexological and discovered that he was highly reactive and had many areas of sensitivity. I also taught him communication skills and touching techniques.

Bob gradually overcame his performance anxiety and got better at achieving and maintaining an erection. In our sixth session, Bob and I had intercourse, and he finally lost his virginity. This was a huge victory, but one problem persisted. He had delayed ejaculation. This is not uncommon for men who struggle with anxiety. Bob couldn't come when he was inside of me or when I stimulated him with my hand or mouth. He could only bring himself to orgasm by masturbating after I had come.

During our last session I encouraged Bob to continue with the exercises he had learned during our time together. I told him, truthfully, that in time I thought he would be able to ejaculate while having intercourse. Then I went into the bathroom to shower and he followed me.

Bob called me the day after our final session to tell me he would pick me up next Wednesday for our photo outing to the University of California's Botanical Garden. Since Bob was no longer a current client it was easier to give myself permission to date him. When he was my client, it had been difficult to come to terms with what was unfolding on a personal level.

Like therapists, surrogates are supposed to avoid personal entanglements with clients. But I felt such a deep connection with Bob that I couldn't ignore it. He was unassuming, bright, and thoughtful. I could talk to him, the way I could talk to Michael, except that I didn't have to contend with an outsized ego or the chronic fear that I somehow wasn't enough. I didn't see how anyone could be hurt by what we were doing.

When Wednesday arrived, I packed up my camera and waited for Bob at my home. Michael, who only worked sporadically, lay on our couch reading a book and when Bob rang the doorbell he let him in. I came out of the bedroom and found them chatting.

"Nice day for a visit to the Botanical Garden," Michael said.

"Yeah, I'm hoping to get some good shots. Great light today."

"I see you two have met," I said.

"Well, I'll let you two go," Michael said and extended his hand to Bob.

It had been in one of our post-session conversations that I had told Bob about my open marriage and that I had recently broken up with my previous lover. Given the work I do he suspected that my marriage was not of the Ozzie and Harriet variety, but the more I got to know Bob the more I wanted him to know the particulars of my arrangement with Michael. If a personal relationship was in the cards for us he had to know that exclusivity would not be part of it—at least for the foreseeable future. While I wasn't ready to admit it, I was starting to imagine a life without Michael to be at least possible, if not desirable.

Bob's reaction was what I expected. He was nonjudgmental, curious, and accepting. He had an endearing quality of being open—even innocent—while still being worldly. It was one of the things I was coming to love about him.

Seeing Michael and Bob side-by-side was an interesting experience for me. I had always been attracted to men with large physiques and Michael was in that category. Bob, on the other hand, was more compact and wiry. And their personalities stood in sharp contrast too. Michael was cocksure about everything. He was a hedonist who always wanted things on his own terms. He felt compelled to foist his opinion into every conversation. C'mon Michael, you're not delivering the Sermon on the Mount, I sometimes found myself thinking when he bloviated about one thing or another. Yes, he was a smart man, but his pontificating was starting to sound pompous and pedantic, and some people found him abrasive. Although Bob was much less sure of himself, and felt uncomfortable in social gatherings, he was much more present emotionally. There was an honesty and sincerity about him that was lacking in Michael. Being with him was more of a shared experience. And our bodies fit together perfectly. Sex with him was sweeter and more intimate than any I had experienced, even with Michael. Bob still suffered from delayed ejaculation and he could only come by masturbating himself after intercourse, but his performance anxiety was firmly a thing of the past. We both hoped that one day he would be able to climax inside of me. It was particularly important for Bob because he saw it as the final hurdle to achieving the kind of intimacy he had pined for all of his adult life.

As Bob and I drove up the Berkeley hills, the August air got warmer as we ascended. Bob parked just outside of the garden and we slung our cameras around our necks. We walked to one of its main paths where red rhododendron, yellow pansies, maroon-speckled white peonies, and a tapestry of other flowers vied for our attention. It was a clear day and the spectacular explosion of color made even a novice photographer like me eager to snap some pictures.

For someone who didn't know an f-stop from a shortstop, I soon found myself beginning to comprehend some of photography's basic concepts and terminology, such as shutter speed, aperture, focal length, and depth of field. It was clear Bob was enjoying our first outing together, and I was grateful for the gentle and patient manner in which he demystified my new camera.

Of all the experimental shots I took that afternoon, the two most memorable are of Bob walking on his hands down a narrow path, and standing on an arch bridge smiling back at me. The first showed his playfulness; the second his kindness.

Although I didn't realize it at the time, I was entering into a new phase of my life, with one foot each in very disparate worlds. The seeds of confusion had been sown, a new emotional landscape lay before me. I soon found myself on a passionate roller coaster, loving all my time spent with Bob and yet still wanting to make my marriage with Michael work.

Bob and I adopted a regular routine of seeing each other about once a week. We went to plays, movies, and museums. There were a few more photography lessons and lots of long hikes. It was all fun, but I think I was happiest when we just hung out, made love, and talked. Sometimes Bob looked at me with such love and affection in his eyes that I would get teary. Maybe love was simpler and sweeter than I had ever imagined.

Bob had season tickets to a few local theater companies and five months after our first date we made a plan to see *She Loves Me*, a romantic musical about two coworkers who don't get along well in person, but fall in love via anonymous letters. Late in the morning of the chilly December day that we were set to see the play I went to Bob's house and we had one of our leisurely afternoons full of love-making and conversation.

We both got so lost in the fun of the day that it came as a shock to suddenly realize that curtain time was only ninety minutes away. Hours had gone by as we lost ourselves in exuberant and blissful sex that had brought me to orgasm a number of times. We planned to have dinner before the show, but Bob was insatiable. We still had to shower and get dressed, and we could always put off dinner until after the play.

I was expecting the wonderful, but what I got was the sublime. With both our eyes and limbs locked in a passionate embrace and our hair and bodies slick with sweat, Bob and I climaxed together for the first time. It was the first time Bob had been able to come while having intercourse. The metamorphosis was complete. Now Bob not only had overcome his inability to get an erection, but his issue with delayed ejaculation.

As with so many men who struggle with this problem, his first orgasm inside a partner occurred totally unexpectedly when he was free of worry and concerns, making love with someone he both loved and trusted.

As Bob and I sat through the show that night watching the main characters, Georg and Amalia, unwittingly falling for each other, we held hands and exchanged loving glances. The music was beautiful, the lyrics clever, and the acting fabulous. Launching a relationship with a former client was risky, but our paths crossed, the moment was right, and the risk paid off in spades.

12.

a second family

As we began the 1980s, Michael and I were as close to monogamous as we would ever come. The first few years after we had opened
our marriage were a time of intense experimentation for both of us,
but eventually we traded extracurricular dalliances for regular and
reliable outside relationships. Mine was with Bob, and Michael's was
with someone he'd met in 1976 at SFSI.

Meg wasn't Michael's type. He usually fell for Rubenesque sorts
whose personalities were as voluptuous as their bodies. He loved curvy,
outspoken, fun-loving women. Meg was short and slight. She wore
her blonde hair close-cropped and had a tomboyish quality about her.
An avid biker and runner, she had a taut, muscular body with little
extra in the way of padding. She was also quiet and pensive. When
I first met her I thought she would be just another one of Michael's
flings that would fizzle soon enough.

I had made a certain peace with our arrangement. There were
even moments when our parallel lives seemed to strike a comfortable

equilibrium. Michael and I could enjoy outside lovers and still honor our primary commitment to our children and the family we had created. At times I felt vindicated because of it, like I had proved my parents and their generation wrong. "See," I wanted to say, "I broke all the rules and came out on top." I had a career I loved, plenty of loyal friends, and, despite its eccentricity, a marriage that had lasted longer than many people had predicted. Overall, I was proud of how Michael and I had forged our own way in life, jettisoning convention and tradition that had outlived its usefulness and holding tight to what mattered.

Most important, my children were happy and healthy. Michael continued to be a loving father who built a strong and ongoing rapport with both Jessica and Eric. I didn't know many kids who could discuss their thoughts, feelings, worries, and dreams with their father the way mine could. I loved how Michael listened—really listened—respectfully and attentively to them. I don't wish every woman could have a husband like Michael, but I do wish every child could have a father like him.

My feelings about our open marriage remained complicated. I was never happy to share Michael with other women, and I felt a pang of jealousy whenever he left to see Meg. At the same time, my outside relationships enriched my life so much that I felt something like gratitude to Michael for freeing me enough to enjoy them without guilt or deception.

The only danger now was that someone would eventually want more than what a married couple with children could give to a secondary relationship. Emotions and attachments had to be managed, gauged just right to fit into the scheme we had constructed. At the center lay Michael, me, and the kids. Other relationships orbited around us, and it could all work out so long as everyone on the periphery stayed happy there.

It was a cool fall day in 1978 when I first found out that Meg no longer was. She asked that Michael and I meet her at her apartment in Berkeley on a Saturday morning. It was earlier than I usually left the house on a weekend, but we had planned a busy day with the kids, and I wanted to get our meeting out of the way. I smelled homemade waffles and coffee as soon as I walked into her tiny, one-bedroom flat. If the circumstances had been different, my appetite probably would have perked up. As it was, when Meg handed me a plate of food and a mug of coffee I knew they would go to waste.

Meg's eyes were rimmed with red and she looked like she hadn't slept.

"How are you, Meg?" I asked.

"I'm fine."

By force of habit I almost said, "Good, thanks," but stopped myself when I realized she hadn't asked how I was.

We sat in her living room and only Michael started eating.

"I know this is awkward, but I needed to—to—"

Meg burst into tears. Michael put his fork down and handed her a tissue.

"What are you people doing?" she said, her voice breaking.

"What do you mean?" I asked.

"Do you know what I had to do, Cheryl?"

I stared at her blankly. I had no idea what she was talking about.

"I had to have an abortion, Michael got me pregnant and I had to have an abortion."

Michael got her pregnant? I assumed he was taking precautions. He chose me because he thought I would make a good mother and he always said the only reason to get married was to have kids. "Kids need two loving, involved parents." I couldn't count how many times I had heard him say that. Surely, he understood that he wouldn't be able to be a good father to two families at the same time. Was this just a slip up?

Michael put his head in his hands.

"Meg, I'm sorry you had to do that, but—"

"Do you two understand how you toy with people?"

I felt bad for Meg, but at the same time I was angry. She was an adult who had gone into the relationship with Michael knowing that he was a married man with two kids. Yes, it was an open marriage, but a marriage nonetheless. He had responsibilities to me and his children that came first. No one lied to her. She didn't enter the tryst under false pretenses. There was no bait and switch. Besides, who did she think would support a child? Michael didn't have a job. I was the sole provider for my family. Meg earned a meager income as a teacher. And why in the world weren't they using birth control?

"Do you? Do you get that?" Meg said.

"Wait a minute. How old are you?" I shot back. "You're a grown woman. You knew what you were getting into. I'm sorry you've been hurt, Meg, but Michael was straight with you from the beginning."

Meg continued to weep. I moved my food around my plate, and Michael stared down as though he was trying to decode a cypher in the rug beneath him.

"It's not right," Meg sobbed.

Michael got up and put his hand on Meg's back. She hugged him and he rocked her in his arms while he looked at me, an apology in his eyes. I was seething and couldn't wait to get Michael alone. I collected the plates and coffee cups, brought them into the kitchen, washed and dried them, and then washed a few other plates that were in the sink. When I returned to the living room Meg had calmed down enough for us to make a graceful exit.

"What the hell is going on?" I demanded the minute I slammed the car door shut. "How did she get pregnant? Aren't you using birth control?"

"She's on the Pill, but you know it's not 100 percent effective. We were just unlucky. What can I do about it?" Michael said.

"I'll tell you what you can do about it. Wear a rubber. Get a vasectomy. Have her get a diaphragm. Don't rely just on the Pill. Make it 100 percent, Michael."

"I know. I know. We'll figure out something. It won't happen again. I promise."

I believed him. Outside relationships were okay; outside families were not. We both knew that.

I didn't see Meg again until nearly a year later, in October 1979. By this time my relationship with Bob was going strong, and I believed that the boundaries had been made sufficiently clear to Meg—and Micheal—at our uncomfortable breakfast. The day she came by I was on the phone chatting with my brother, who still lived in New England, when the doorbell rang. I put down the phone and when I opened the door I found Meg standing on our front porch. We looked at each other for a moment, both of us slightly surprised. Finally, I said hello. She told me she was there to pick up a turntable that Michael had stored for her in our basement. To my relief, I heard our bedroom door open and Michael soon rescued me from the awkward moment.

I picked up the phone again and talked to my brother for close to an hour. A few minutes before we hung up I looked out the front window and saw Meg unlock her car door and Michael load the turntable into the backseat. Something looks different about her, I thought. Then it occurred to me that she was wearing overalls. This was an odd choice for Meg, who normally wore athletic clothes. Spandex leggings and long T-shirts were a virtual uniform for her.

Weird, I thought, but what did I care? I had better things to do than ponder Meg's bizarre sartorial choice.

In 1980, my daughter was fourteen and my son was eleven. They were in the angst-soaked preadolescent and teen years and I was determined to see them through it with the sensitivity and compassion that I didn't get from my parents. I tried to be the relaxed, sensitive, helpful mother that mine never was to me. I wanted my kids to be able to come to me with anything and to never fear my anger.

I still harbored anger toward my parents, but I'd tried to mend the rift with them, for both myself and my children. Mom and Dad loved their grandkids and I wanted my daughter and son to have as many adoring adults in their lives as possible. I had paid a heavy price for carrying around anger toward them all those years and letting it go was something I gradually worked through in therapy and in life. At least twice a year I returned to Salem for a visit. My parents' relationship with Michael had thawed some, but not enough for him to want to join me on most of those trips. In early 1980, I decided I would go back to Massachusetts for a visit in May.

Shortly after I confirmed the dates of my trip I got a call from my friend Brendan, a lawyer with a thriving practice in San Francisco. He had reservations he had to cancel for a weekend at Yosemite's Ahwahnee Hotel, complete with dinner in their stunning dining room on both nights. They were for early May. Did Michael and I want to take them?

The Ahwahnee Hotel is an architectural marvel that combines a number of classical and modern styles. It has a wonderful eatery that offers breathtaking views of the Yosemite wilderness. On our own Michael and I would never have been able to afford a weekend there, but thanks to Brendan, we suddenly had a chance to get away in style. Michael looked forward to it as much as I did.

I always faced a visit back home with a certain amount of anxiety, but now I knew that just a week before I left I could relax and rejuvenate in the middle of one of the most tranquil and beautiful places on earth. I decided that I would treat myself to a new dress for dinner at the Ahwahnee. It had been a long time since I had indulged in an extravagance that was all mine. Unlike most of my clothes, which came from secondhand shops, I would be the first one to wear my new ensemble.

I woke up early one Saturday morning in February and went into San Francisco. I spent the day at department stores and boutiques searching for just the right dress for my getaway. Sure, it was early. The trip was still months away, but I was overdue for a splurge. I finally found a green, sleeveless, silk dress with a cinched waste and hand-beading around its scalloped neckline. I tried it on and turned around in the mirror to see myself from all angles. It was perfect. I would look as sophisticated as anyone else at the exclusive Ahwahnee. It meant parting with $200 I had scraped together in the last few months, but it wasn't often that I got a chance for a lavish trip and I was going to make the most of it.

I looked forward to the trip for months. I navigated the hectic schedule of any working mom, reminding myself that my weekend of luxury was drawing closer. Sometimes, after a tough day, I peaked at the dress hanging in the closet or tried it on and reminded myself that I would soon have a break from my workaday life. I was also looking forward to some much-needed time alone with Michael. We rarely got a chance to be together without the kids, and when we did we reacquainted ourselves with the reasons we fell in love. Lately it felt like we were drifting apart, and I hoped that our jaunt would rekindle the intimacy between us.

On the Thursday before we were set to leave for Yosemite I took the afternoon off from work. I still needed to pick up my tickets at the travel agency for my trip back East later that month, and I wanted plenty of time to pack. I stood in my bedroom and looked into the open mouth of my suitcase. I was trying to figure out how to fold the elegant dress I had bought so that it wouldn't wrinkle. I decided not to take any chances. Instead of packing it away I would keep it on its hanger and lay it out in the backseat of the car. All I had to do was cover it with the garment bag that I knew I had somewhere and the dress would arrive in pristine condition.

At the time Michael and I had a space-saver bed that was built atop a set of drawers. Michael made it shortly after we had moved into our house. Even though I didn't like it at first, I had to admit that in our glorified closet of a bedroom having a dresser and bed in one made sense. I looked through the drawers on my side of the bed, but the garment bag was nowhere to be found. I walked over to Michael's side. What a slob, I thought as I looked around. As usual, his side of the room was littered with candy wrappers, newspapers, and old tissues. A half-finished bottle of Dr. Pepper stood next to the lamp on the nightstand. I had long ago given up trying to keep his area neat. I slid open the top drawer and pulled out the sweaters and T-shirts that were in it. That's when I saw the letters that lay at the bottom of the drawer.

There were about twenty-five of them, all from Meg to Michael, postmarked from a city in the Pacific Northwest. I took them out and laid them on the bed. Then I arranged them in chronological order, my heart pounding and my hands shaking. I felt like I wanted to run. I had to read these letters, but I had to get out of there to go pick up my tickets too. My skin felt as confining as a prison cell. I have to get my tickets, I thought. Then impulse took over. I grabbed an old tote bag, gathered the letters together so I wouldn't break their order, and shoved them into it.

I drove several blocks and pulled into a parking garage just outside of the travel agency. I opened the tote bag and fingered the pile of letters. My limbs felt leaden and my jaw ached from squeezing it so hard. One by one, I read through the missives that detailed Meg's pregnancy. She wrote of how excited her parents were to have a grand-child on the way; about doctor's visits and potential names; and she told Michael how much she missed him and their mind-blowing sex, the sex that gave her the child she so wanted. "The doctor says it could happen any day now," she wrote in one of her later dispatches.

It's hard to describe the cascade of emotions that seized me while I read. Anxiety, rage, and desperation took hold. It was the emotional equivalent of the car wreck we had suffered on our way out West. These were feelings of grotesque intensity and I could no more think them away than I could will away the physics of the car crash. Both forces were too strong for me to escape.

I sat in the car for close to an hour, trying to compose myself enough to go into the travel agency and get my plane ticket for Boston. I took out my wallet and counted out the money for my trip. I did that two more times just to forestall having to see anyone. I put the money back into its envelope and stepped out of the car. As I walked toward the exit a tall man loped toward me. I think it was at this time that I dropped my money and that the man must have scooped it up and took off with it. All I know is that when I got into the travel agency I was missing $400.

When I arrived home I was thankful for two things: First, that I hadn't had an accident, and second, that the house was still empty. I got into bed and cried. This betrayal was like none other I had experienced. I cried for many reasons. I was furious, humiliated, and hurt. What made the pain bottomless was that Michael had now obliterated the one thing that made our marriage meaningful. He was no longer having kids only with me. Apparently, he thought Meg would do just as well as a mother, and the one claim to exclusivity that I could make was gone. Was our whole marriage a farce? I flashed back to that October day when I'd seen Meg in overalls. She was pregnant. That's why she wore them, I realized with a swift and awful clarity.

I didn't know exactly how I would act on this new information, but I wasn't going to sit quietly on it. This was too earth-shattering for me to feign ignorance. I just didn't know how I would begin the conversation, and as much as I insisted to myself that I had to stay cool, I knew I wouldn't.

I had to pull myself together. The kids would be home soon and Michael probably would be too. I dried my eyes and blew my nose, hoping it would halt my tears. I folded up the letters and slid them back in their envelopes. I placed them back in the drawer, whimpering the whole time.

When I heard the door open I knew it was Jessica and Eric coming home from school.

"Hello?" Eric called.

I ran into the bathroom.

I took a deep breath and yelled, "In the bathroom."

I tried, but I couldn't mask the tears in my voice.

"Are you okay?" Eric called back.

"Yes—fine. I just took a little nap. Getting into the shower."

I turned on the water, stripped off my clothes, and took my second shower of the day. It was the only way I could buy some time and pull myself together so that my kids didn't see the hysterical mess I had become.

After dinner Michael still wasn't home. I got into bed and tried to read, but spent most of the evening crying. At around ten I heard him come through the door. I switched off the light, rolled over, and pretended to be asleep.

I listened to Michael rummage around the kitchen and flip on the TV. Soon he came into the bedroom. He has no idea I know, I thought. I watched his dark shape as he pulled off his jeans and put on a pair of sweatpants. I felt like a voyeur watching a stranger.

Late the next morning Michael and I packed up the car, kissed Jessica and Eric goodbye, and started the three-and-half-hour drive to the Ahwahnee. Michael was at the wheel. He turned onto I-580 and blended into the freeway traffic.

"So, I'm leaving for Salem soon," I said.

"Yeah," Michael answered.

"I'll be flying across country. It's a big trip. Anything could happen. What if the plane crashed? Is there anything you'd want to tell me?"

"What? What are you talking about?"

"You know. If I were to die suddenly, is there anything you'd want me to know?"

"No. Of course not."

We stopped for lunch about two hours later, and when we got back in the car we listened to music and I thought about how I would try to pry Michael's secret from him.

We arrived at the Ahwahnee at around four o'clock, both of us hungry and tired from the trip. We checked into our room and rested for a little while. Then I took a shower, put on the dress I had bought for the occasion, styled my hair, and put on some lipstick and mascara. I looked in the mirror at myself and thought about how much I had uncovered since I had bought the smart, green silk dress. I felt foolish for buying it now. It was the action of someone happily buzzing along, oblivious to the disaster gathering around her. When I stepped out of the bathroom Michael smiled at me. "You look so pretty," he said. I forced a smile and grabbed my purse.

Michael put on a sport coat and we made our way down to the restaurant. The Ahwahnee dining room was spectacular. It had high ceilings and giant windows that looked out onto the lush scenery. I would have really liked this, I said to myself. We ordered dinner and a bottle of wine. Soon I was a little tipsy and I fished again to see if I could get Michael to talk.

"Are you sure there's nothing you want to tell me? Imagine this is your last chance to come clean."

"What do you mean? What's going on with you?"

"I just think we should have total honesty with each other and you never know what will happen."

It was taking every bit of strength I had to keep from confronting him. I was so angry I wanted to stand up and scream, I know what's going on!

"I have nothing to tell you."

The next morning I decided I would stop trying to pull Michael's secret out of him. He wasn't going to confess, so if I wanted a reckoning I would have to initiate it directly. Trying to finesse his secret out of him was a lost cause. I was still seething, and it was going to take a lot of effort to keep my emotions under control.

We hiked for most of the day. I pushed myself physically as hard as could to try to release some of the anger and anxiety that churned in me. Michael had gained weight over the years and he breathed so hard that he couldn't carry on a conversation as we trooped along the strenuous trail. This was a huge relief. I didn't think I could bear to make everyday chatter at this point. When we circled back to the mouth of trail, Michael and I were both ready for a rest and we headed back to the room.

We ate dinner in the dining room again, and even though I had a few glasses of wine I restrained myself from probing Michael for a confession. We headed back to our room. I made love with Michael passionately. In my mind I was thinking about how I wanted to remind him of what he would miss if I weren't in his life. I was exhausted from holding back my emotions the whole trip. Even if Michael would never know it, this gave me a way to express them—if only in a passive-aggressive way. When we were done, Michael fell asleep in my arms. I lay awake for a few hours and then finally drifted off.

I woke up the next morning just as the sun began painting the sky a dusty pink. I looked at the ceiling and for a moment mourned my ignorance. What a delight this weekend would have been if I still had it. What was I going to do? This was a secret I wouldn't keep, a juggernaut I couldn't sidestep. I propped myself up on my elbow and stared at Michael. His chest rose and fell and he snored slightly. I watched him for a few minutes. Then he opened his eyes and looked at me.

"What? What's going on? What are you doing?" he said.

"I know, Michael. I know about the baby."

His mouth hung open.

"What baby?" he said.

"You know what baby, Michael. I know Meg's preg—"

My voice cracked and the tears flooded out of me.

"I don't know what to do with this," I whimpered.

Michael said nothing.

"How do you think you've made me feel, Michael?"

"I thought you wouldn't mind," he said.

What? He thought I wouldn't mind? This was last thing I expected him to say. It wasn't just the wrong answer, it was an outlandish one. How could he think I wouldn't mind? I half-expected the *Twilight Zone* theme song to kick in. Reality had been turned on its head.

"Who are you? Who do you think I am? I've trusted that you know me better than anyone in this world, and you don't know me at all."

"I thought you'd be okay with it."

"What?" I yelled. "What made you think I would be okay with it? What was your plan? When were you going to tell me?"

"Well, I thought I would wait until the child was a teenager."

"What? Are you kidding?"

Michael looked away.

"I mean are you fucking serious? We'd be together all these years and then I'd open the door one day to a mysterious teenager who would turn out to be your child. And then what? You'd introduce me and we'd just go on as normal?"

"Cheryl, it doesn't matter. You're my wife, not Meg. She had the baby a few weeks ago, and I wasn't even there. I was with you."

Was this supposed to comfort me? Was it Michael's twisted way of telling me that I was special to him?

"If it didn't matter why did you keep it a secret?" I demanded.

Michael took a deep breath and put his head in his hand.

"What difference does it make? You're my wife, not Meg."

I felt like I was going to vomit. I stood up and walked to the window. I pushed the curtain aside and stared out into the wilderness. What had seemed so beautiful to me before now looked like a mess, a tangled, incoherent welter that swallowed people up and hid all sorts of danger.

"She had the baby. What was it, Michael? Do you have another son or another daughter?" I asked, still staring out the window.

"A girl. She had a girl."

I turned around and faced him.

"How could you let this happen? You promised after the first accident that you would be more careful."

"Meg really wanted a child and she's getting older. She told me I owed it to her after she had the abortion, but, Cheryl, it's not going to involve me. I won't be in their lives."

"You owed it to her? You didn't tell her that was crazy? And you're okay with having nothing to do with this child?"

I certainly wasn't okay with it, far from it.

"She's with her mother. Meg has a big family. They support her. They were happy when they found out she was pregnant. The child will be cared for."

I don't know how I didn't fall over. The man I'd considered a model father, who had talked with such earnestness about how children need the attention and affection of both of their parents was now telling me that he planned to walk out on his responsibility for his child.

"No, Michael. If we're going to stay together you're not going to abandon your child. You're going to spend time with the baby. You'll visit two or three times a year. How can you imagine your child not knowing her father? And one more thing: This is it. You're not going to fuck any more women. Not now that you've made another family."

"Okay. Okay. I can make this work," Michael said.

Michael was taking it all in too easily. It was almost as if my demands really didn't require any great shift in what was already in the works.

"You don't have a choice now."

I said all of this as if what I wanted mattered to him. The crazy thing was that despite it all I still loved Michael. I had grown enough to be able to conceive of a life without him, but not enough to want it. In many ways Michael was a scoundrel. I came to see this more and more not just by his actions, but because of something I had been doing for the last year now: comparing him to Bob.

Bob remained the same steadfast, supportive, sweet man I had fallen for a year ago. I saw him shortly after the Ahwahnee trip. I told him about Michael's new family and he comforted me while I cried enough tears to float the *Queen Mary*. Bob's only concern was for me. He didn't bash Michael and he didn't try to turn the situation to his advantage. Another man might have spied an opportunity and prodded me to dump my husband, who, even within the context of an open marriage, could be called a philanderer. Not Bob. He simply didn't think in opportunistic terms, especially with me. Had I decided to leave Michael he would have supported me, but I also knew that he would stay by my side even if I didn't. He simply loved me and wanted me to be happy. When I shared the devastating news with him he helped me into bed and stroked my forehead as I wept. I felt awfully sorry for myself, but when I dried my tears and saw Bob's concerned face staring down at me, I also wondered how I managed to get so lucky.

13.

what if?: bradley

Several years after Michael turned my personal world upside down, I had an experience at work which, for the first time, truly frightened me.

Bradley came to me from Pamela, a local therapist who I had worked with in the past.

He was not a typical client. His pathology was much more profound and infinitely more disturbing than that of any other client. Bradley had recently been released from prison. He had served a five-year sentence for molesting a seven-year-old girl. Before I agreed to see him, I had a long discussion with Pamela about what our work would entail. Pamela was working in conjunction with a colleague who specialized in treating pedophilia. They were testing the notion that they could, with the help of surrogacy and other treatment, redirect the sexual urges of men like Bradley to adult women. Bradley was not the first client with whom they had tried this approach.

There were a few others and there had been encouraging signs with some of them. Pamela hoped these cases would lay the groundwork for a breakthrough treatment that would ultimately serve to make children safer.

It was not easy to make the choice to work with Bradley. I admired Pamela's efforts to rehabilitate someone who had served his sentence and was reentering society, changed or not. On the other hand, I would be working with, and be vulnerable to, someone who was guilty of one of the most hideous crimes a human being can commit. As a parent, I was sickened by what Bradley had done, yet, as a parent, I also felt if I could play some role in protecting children I should. I decided to take Bradley on as a client. Maybe it sounds naïve or idealistic, but I thought if my skills as a surrogate could help professionals like Pamela develop a treatment model that could ameliorate this dangerous disorder, then I needed to step up to the plate.

The role of compassion in the surrogacy process cannot be overstated. I infuse my work with it. If I didn't, I doubt I would be able to be effective at what I do. With Bradley, I would have to make an extra conscious and concerted effort to remain compassionate. That is, of course, not to say that I was remotely comfortable with what he had done. I had to struggle mightily to leave my fear behind and approach Bradley with the same openness I would give to any other client. It was difficult, but I did it because if I take on a client I commit to doing the best I can to help him resolve his problem, and my best comes from a base of compassion, not contempt.

When I scheduled the appointment with Bradley over the phone he wasn't difficult or defensive, but I had the feeling that he was just going along, just doing what he had been told to do.

In the days leading up to our first meeting, I did my best to manage my fear and trepidation. I had to remind myself frequently of the ultimate goal of this work. Pamela and I had another discussion about Bradley the day before my appointment with him. We talked about how I would alter my protocol to suit his treatment. We decided that given the intensive and customized therapy he was receiving from

Pamela, I wouldn't delve as deeply into his childhood and early sexual history as I did with other clients.

Like many pedophiles, he had been sexually abused as a child by a close family member. Pamela had been working with him for about three months. He complied with treatment, he reported to his parole officer when he was required to, and there was no indication that he had reoffended. Bradley was living near his sister and holding down a steady job as a technician at a local lab. He seemed to be doing all the right things, yet Pamela hadn't seen him express much insight or remorse. Could someone like Bradley really be rewired and transformed, or was the pathology too insidious, too deep to be reached by surrogacy or any of the therapy modalities currently available?

I scheduled Bradley's appointment for the morning, hoping to get it over with early in the day and limit the number of anxious hours that would inevitably lead up to the appointment. I got up earlier than normal and did some of the invaluable breathing and relaxation exercises I had learned in my surrogacy training. By the time he arrived, I had tamed most of my apprehension and was determined to do the best I could with him.

When I opened the door and saw this slight, dark-haired man, however, I felt a chill run down my spine. He was, in a word, creepy. My fingers started to tingle and my breathing sped up. I felt like a cord was being cinched around my shoulders and chest. I started talking immediately to pull myself out of my fear. "Thank you for coming," I said. Bradley nodded and stepped into my office. He had ruddy skin and oily black hair that looked like it was unwashed and maybe recently dyed.

I asked a few perfunctory questions. He told me a bit about his limited experience with women, which involved failure to maintain an erection and difficulty staying in a relationship for more than a few weeks. The last time he'd had a girlfriend was eight years ago, when he was twenty-two. Bradley had a vacant, impervious quality I'd never encountered in anyone else. I described the surrogacy process to him and explained how it involved a gradual deepening of intimacy and regular feedback.

Then it was time to go to the bedroom. I felt my stomach gather into a knot, so I took a deep breath while I led Bradley down the hall. Once we'd undressed I noticed that his skin had a purplish tinge to it. I don't want him on my sheets, I thought, even though I knew that's where we were headed. As we lay next to each other, I started working through various relaxation exercises, as much for myself as for him. I asked him to close his eyes and to take some deep breaths. He ignored me and started chattering about the drive over, the food in prison, his upcoming fishing trip, his growing dislike of his boss, and any number of other random topics. Every time I tried to encourage him to quietly focus on his body and take deep breaths he would stop talking for a few seconds and then return to rambling.

Lying beside him was difficult, and for the first and only time in my career, I decided to omit Spoon Breathing. I simply couldn't stand to be that close to him. We began Sensual Touch. I knelt down on the floor and started touching Bradley's feet. His toenails were too long and had crescents of grime beneath them. A voice in my mind screamed, Get the hell out of here! If only I could. By this time I had moved my office into my home. If I fled I would have to leave Bradley there. I continued up Bradley's body. His skin was cold and clammy and the backs of his knees were crisscrossed with spider veins. He smelled of sweat and stale cigarettes.

Bradley had not stopped yammering and as I made my way up his body he started talking about things that made my flesh crawl. He told me about Gina, the child he had molested. She was the seven-year-old daughter of a former employer.

"Bradley, it's important for you to try to concentrate on your body right now. Just follow my hands and notice what kind of sensations you have as I touch you."

"Gina betrayed me," he said, totally ignoring my latest plea for quiet. "Theresa would never do that."

"Theresa?" I asked.

"My neighbor with the blonde curls," he said.

My hands were on the backs of his sinewy thighs.

"Theresa comes over after school to look at me in my special shorts. The ones she can see me in."

I took my hands off of him and sat back on my knees.

"She loves watching me get bigger and bigger and giggles when I spill out of my shorts. Yesterday I touched her hair for the first time. Pretty soon it will be time to invite her in. Not yet, though."

I flashed on Pamela telling me there was no sign Bradley had reoffended. Why was he telling me this? Didn't he realize I was obligated to tell the authorities? Didn't he know I would? Then I started panicking. What if he attacked me? If I had to save my life, I'd knee him in the crotch with all of my might, but would it be enough? What if he overpowered me? What if he was quicker than me? No one was around, so my screams would go unheard. What if he sprung up and grabbed me around the throat? My fear for myself may have been a little misplaced because Bradley showed no signs of agitation. In fact, he seemed no more affected than if he had just rattled off his street address.

I slowly stood up, began dressing, and asked Bradley to do the same. I told him we had come to the end of our first session. "Bradley," I said, "it was nice to meet you. I'm not sure if surrogacy work will help you with the issues you're dealing with, so let me have a talk with Pamela before we schedule our next session."

He zippered up his pants, put on his denim jacket, and headed out. I watched him get into his car and drive off. I misdialed Pamela's phone number twice, and when I said hello my voice sounded hollow.

"Cheryl?" Pamela asked.

"Yes. It's me. Sorry. I just finished my session with Bradley. He has to be stopped." I told Pamela what Bradley had revealed to me and asked if she would call the police, or if I should. Pamela promptly hung up with me and made the call.

My experience with Bradley was without a doubt the most frightening incident of my career. After my hair-raising experience with him I took a few days off. I was reminded of how vulnerable I am in the work that I do. I was so accustomed to thinking of my clients as the ones taking the risks and gathering the courage it took to make change that I rarely thought about the physical danger my job could pose.

One morning that week, as I sipped coffee in my kitchen, I decided to go through my file cabinet that was jammed with client files. I opened the top drawer and pulled out as many as I could carry over to the sofa. I started thumbing through them. There had been so many successes, so many kind, decent people who had come to see me because they wanted to have deeper intimacy, love, and connection with a current or future partner. These were my clients. This was exactly what I needed to put the ordeal with Bradley into perspective. I was reminded, again, why I do this work.

14.

a frightening new disease

....

"**H**ow are you different from a prostitute?" It's high on the list of the most common questions put to me. Sometimes it's asked sheepishly; other times it's an accusation disguised as an inquiry. In the early part of my career I struggled with how to best answer it. I was clear on the difference, but I didn't know how much detail to go into about what I did with clients and why a profession like mine was necessary.

Steven Brown, a male surrogate I'd become close friends with in the late '70s, solved that problem for me by crafting an analogy that I still use today. When you go to a prostitute it's like going to a restaurant. You choose from the menu, you eat, and when you leave the proprietor hopes you will return and tell your friends. Seeing a surrogate is like going to culinary school. You learn the recipes, develop your skills in the kitchen, broaden your palate, and then go out into the world with your newfound knowledge. If all goes well, you create delicious meals for select dining partners again and again. "That's exactly right. In a way I'm more Julia Child than Xavier

Hollander," I said when Steven first shared this with me. Call me the happy cooker.

Steven was one of only a few male surrogates and his clients were primarily gay men. I liked him from the first time we met. With his dark hair, angular face, and tall, lean body, he had no problem finding sex partners. He and I dished about our lovers and laughed about exploits. We discussed our work as well, and this helped both of us to become better surrogates. You can't swap work stories with the other PTA moms when you're a surrogate, so I was thankful to have a confidant who shared my profession and could appreciate its challenges and rewards. Steven and I leaned on each other in the way true friends can. Sometimes he would half-jokingly say we should get married, but I already had two husbands.

On October 31, 1981, Bob and I drove to Reno and got married. The ceremony took place in the City Hall building and was conducted by a Justice of the Peace. She read a Native American wedding blessing that seemed like it was written for us. "Now you will feel no rain, for each of you will be the shelter for each other. Now you will feel no cold, for each of you will be the warmth for the other," it began. This was the kind of mutual care that sustained our partnership. "Treat yourselves and each other with respect, and remind yourselves often of what brought you together. Give the highest priority to the tenderness, gentleness, and kindness that your connection deserves," it went on. I had no doubt that this would be the creed that governed our future together. When she was done with the prayer, Bob and I exchanged rings and walked out of the chapel into the crisp autumn air.

We checked into Harrah's hotel and had some of the best sex of our lives. We were now husband and wife, and our lovemaking was a celebration of our deepened union. It was a four-poster honeymoon. I felt the kind of joy I'd feared I no longer had the capacity for after the events of the last year. I could still love and be loved. Bob and my commitment to each other was unshakable and now it was official— well, sort of. It couldn't be legal because I was still married to Michael.

I didn't care. Bob and I could never have children, as I was infertile and he'd had a vasectomy. So when he asked me if I would marry him, just for us, I said yes because I truly trusted and loved him. The ceremony was never meant to be official in any way, but rather a pledge of personal devotion to each other. Bob explained that he knew that I was the love of his life, and that having me in his life part-time would be more fulfilling than having someone else full-time.

When Michael learned about how I had spent Halloween he was furious, but it didn't matter to me. I had suffered the humiliation of his extramarital family, so as far as I was concerned, if he had a problem with me taking a second husband, that was just too bad. "You're going to have to deal with it, Michael—just like I've had to deal with you having a family with Meg," I declared. Michael made a hasty call to a lawyer friend. His hope, I'm sure, was that he would hear that I had jeopardized our family's financial future. "What if he sues us? He could take everything," Michael roared. Michael never elaborated on what specific legal maneuvering he feared, and I didn't press him. Bob would never do anything of the sort and neither Michael nor I could articulate the legal grounds that he would act on even if he were so inclined. We both knew it was a bid to drum up fear, regret, and guilt in me, and we both knew it wouldn't work. Michael's hollow threat didn't scare me and he quickly dropped it.

Bob's dedication to me never waned. In 1983, Michael tossed another hand grenade at our relationship. Meg was pregnant again. If I was impressed that Bob didn't judge Michael, I was also impressed that he didn't judge me. I wouldn't have blamed him if he demanded to know what was wrong with me. Why did I continue to stay with someone who used my heart as a doormat? Love has its own logic. Bob knew this, and I guess he also knew that the best way he could help was to love me in his own uncompromising way. I had never known such unselfish adoration. Without him, I probably would have concluded that I was fundamentally unlovable, simply not good enough for anyone to devote himself to me. Bob gave me proof to the contrary. But it was still Michael whom I lived with and returned to almost every night.

I wasn't ready to leave Michael. My love for him resembled a law of nature. I didn't choose it any more than I chose to stay firmly planted on the earth by gravity. I couldn't fully explain to myself or anyone else why I loved him, and that scared me. I had warned him that he was going to destroy the love I had for him if he kept hurting me. It wasn't gone, but it had begun to look irrational, and I had started to resent it. Sometimes when I was alone, I sat quietly and tried to imagine returning to the affection I felt for him in the early days. No matter how hard I looked, though, I couldn't glimpse a road back. All I could see was that imagination has its limits.

∾

It wasn't only my personal life that was roiled in the early '80s. Around that time the surrogacy world was rocked with fear about a frightening new disease that filled the media. We weren't sure exactly how it was transmitted and not even a hint of a cure or treatment existed. It affected mostly gay men, but it had been diagnosed in heterosexuals as well. At first Steven knew one person with it, then he knew two, then five, then seven. Fear shot through the San Francisco bathhouses that he and his friends frequented. People talked in grave tones about what was starting to look like an epidemic. It was a wasting syndrome, and its victims were struck with repeated infections, lymphoma, Kaposi's sarcoma, thrush, pneumonia, and other grim conditions. Steven had seen friends go from burly to skeletal as the disease ruthlessly winnowed away their bodies and lives. AIDS had made its terrible debut.

Surrogates and other sex workers were as confused as the general public—probably more scared. In 1983, the news media reported that AIDS had been seen in heterosexual women. Conjecture flew about how the disease was transmitted. Could you get it from kissing? From sharing a cigarette? Was it airborne? Like every surrogate I knew, I was trying to find reliable information and exact truth from the onslaught of rumor and speculation. I was also questioning if I could stay in my profession. I considered suspending my practice. Maybe it was time to look for other work. I had trained as a massage therapist. I supposed I could do that, but what if I touched someone who was sweaty? Could I get AIDS from that? If my worry wasn't going to spiral into panic, I needed information fast.

The CDC issued a statement about the transmission of AIDS in 1983 saying, in part, that AIDS " . . . seems most likely to be caused by an agent transmitted by intimate sexual contact, through contaminated needles, or, less commonly, by percutaneous inoculation of infectious blood or blood products." They also said that there was no evidence that it was spread via air, or that casual contact posed a major risk. The picture became clearer. I could stop worrying that I or my kids would contract AIDS with a handshake or from a cough. Still, I needed a plan to keep myself as safe as possible. Surrogates were starting to leave the profession, and I had decided that I wasn't going to follow them. I loved being a surrogate. It was my life's work and I wasn't going to walk away from it. I pledged to become as educated as I could about AIDS, and to change my practice to limit my vulnerability to it.

In 1984, Steven, a few other Bay Area surrogates and I piled into a van and drove to Palm Springs for the Society for the Scientific Study of Sexuality, or "Quad S" conference, where there would be much talk of AIDS and its transmission. We had gone to these conferences in the past, and while they were always an occasion for serious discussion, they were also festive. It was an opportunity for likeminded people to join together and to catch up with old friends. The days were spent learning, trading notes, and opining on the pressing issues in our field. The nights were for fun. We gathered together for dinner and drinks and the laughing and socializing often stretched into the early morning hours.

That a new era was in store for us couldn't have been more evident at Quad S that year. Even the airy Southern California hotel with its aquamarine color scheme and curved walls couldn't disguise the mood. People were crying and recalling friends and members of our community who had been taken by the scourge that was now upon us. Anxiety was high. These were surrogates and other sex educators, therapists, physicians, and a variety of other professionals. Many of us were reeling from losses and all were confused about how to best advise the people who turned to us for help. Past conferences seemed like a somewhat raucous college reunion. This one seemed more like a memorial service.

It was the first time I remember hearing the term "safe sex," which later gave way to the more accurate "safer sex." Our community may have been mourning, but it also had to become educated at breakneck speed. We were entering a new era in which the old fears of treatable STDs and pregnancy were nothing compared to what we now faced. The takeaway messages from the convention about prevention were unequivocal. Condoms were now a must. For the first time we learned about using dental barriers and non-microwavable plastic wrap for oral contact. If you wanted to stay safe, say goodbye to anonymous, unprotected sex. A new era had been foisted on us and its choices were stark. Our thinking may have been as progressive as ever, but our actions needed to become a lot more conservative.

When I returned to the Bay Area, I enrolled in a class on eroticizing latex at the Institute for the Advanced Study of Human Sexuality in San Francisco. We learned how to turn condoms, dental dams, and other preventative tools into sex toys. In addition to providing us with potentially life-saving information, the class was proof that sex education could be fun. We practiced putting on condoms with our mouths and devised creative ways to have non-penetrative sex. I also learned how to erotically check that a condom stayed in place in the midst of vigorous intercourse. From then on I kept a supply of condoms at my office. Using them is mandatory—and fun. I started modeling not just good, but safer sex.

15.

going oral: kevin

Like many people, I roared with laughter at the *Seinfeld* episode in which Jerry finally shares "the move" with George. It may have been especially funny for me because people sometimes think I teach "techniques" that are sure to please all women (or men). But I don't teach them, and they don't exist. What drives one person wild may have another reaching for the TV remote.

The technique I do teach, however, and that has a proven track record of working, is communication. Sometimes it can be communication about serious underlying issues, but more often it's simply the ability to talk about what feels pleasurable and what doesn't. It's tough for some of us to tactfully tell a partner that we don't like what he or she is doing, and to suggest an alternative. We worry about bruising egos or hurting feelings, and there is a great temptation to avoid discussion that makes us feel awkward. It's comforting to think that not talking about a problem will somehow make it go away, but we all know that doesn't work. It drives whatever the problem is underground where it can fester and mutate into more of an issue than it ever would be out in the open.

Talking honestly and respectfully about what works and what doesn't under the sheets is the best way I know to build an exciting sex life. Many clients have proven this to me, but the one who exemplified it the most was Kevin, who came to see me in the mid-1980s.

Kevin was suffering from what he called "impotence." He had a girlfriend, Diane, whom he loved, but he regularly lost his erection with her. Diane had begun to wonder if he didn't find her attractive, or if he was bored with her, and this drove him to therapy. He didn't understand how he could have such attraction for the wonderful woman in his life and not be able sustain an erection with her. He feared that there was something radically wrong with him, or that he was simply a bad lover whom Diane would eventually trade for a better one.

That Kevin was determined to change was evident at our first session. He had an earnest desire to understand and address his issue. He also had a level of frustration with himself that was at odds with the rational approach he had adopted. He knew self-blame wouldn't fix the problem, but he felt it anyway.

I asked Kevin to talk about why he had come to see me.

"I don't understand, and I've tried to look at it in every way I can," he said.

He took off his wire-rim glasses and placed them on his khaki-covered knee.

"I mean, I love my girlfriend, she turns me on, and yet when we try to have sex, I lose my erection."

Unlike many other clients, Kevin could talk about sex without embarrassment. Words like "erection" are difficult for some clients even to utter, but I couldn't detect any change in his demeanor as he said it.

I asked him if he had experienced this in the past.

"Never. And Diane is the first woman I truly love," he said.

"Do you become partially or completely flaccid when you lose your erection?"

"Completely. It's like I go back to not being aroused at all."

I asked Kevin if there was a pattern to how he and Diane typically made love. Did they start with foreplay, or just jump into it? What kind of touch did they engage in? Who typically initiated sex?

"When we first started seeing each other, I mostly made the first move, but now I'm so scared of failing that I've backed off. For a while Diane was initiating, but now she's scared too. When we were having . . . er . . . trying to have sex, we started with foreplay, which we both love. We French kiss and touch each other all over. Then she goes down on me or I eat her out. That's usually when the problem starts. That's when I lose it, and ruin everything."

"Do you both enjoy oral sex?"

"Yes, I like getting it and giving it, and so does Diane."

Given this, it was curious that the mood typically shifted at this point. It would be important to pay close attention to how Kevin responded when I performed oral sex on him during the Sexological. Maybe this would give us both some clues to what was undermining his sex life.

"Kevin, this isn't your fault, or anyone's fault. We'll try to get a better sense of what's underlying your issue as we work through some exercises, but one thing that will help is if you can try to let go of self-blame. Let's start with you trying to be compassionate with yourself and not seeing this as a failure on your part. Deal?"

"Okay. Deal," Kevin replied, somewhat grudgingly.

I explained Sensual Touch to Kevin and asked him if he was ready to try it.

He stood up. He was a small man, probably no more than five-foot-four. He was trim, except for a small roll of belly fat that barely protruded over his belted waist.

In the bedroom I took off my blouse, pants, and underwear, and invited Kevin to undress and settle into bed.

We started off by lying in spoon position and breathing together. I asked him to lie on his side and bend his legs. Then I snuggled up next to him and put my hand over his abdomen. "Just breathe the way you normally would and I'll follow along," I said.

He took even, easy breaths in and out. I mimicked his breathing and soon we harmonized into a steady rhythm of inhales and exhales. I felt his abdomen gently expand and contract.

"Doing great, Kevin," I said.

In and out, in and out, we continued for several minutes. Then Kevin's breath picked up and his body got warmer.

"How are you doing?" Kevin said he was fine.

I slowly got up and stood by the side of the bed. I could see that Kevin had an erection.

"An erection at this point usually means that you're relaxed, which is the best thing you can be right now. If you're ready, please roll over onto your abdomen in the middle of the bed, but make sure you adjust yourself so you're comfortable," I said.

Kevin slowly rolled over and slipped his hand under his groin to adjust his hardened penis.

I knelt on the floor and took Kevin's feet in my hands. When I pressed on the arches he started to giggle.

"You're ticklish there," I said.

"Sorry."

"That's okay, nothing wrong with it at all. However you react to my touch is okay. I'm going to apply a little more pressure, so it doesn't tickle, but it's okay that it did."

I pressed my thumbs into the arches of Kevin's feet and moved them around in circles.

Kevin's body reacted almost immediately to my touch. As I worked my way up his legs, the tension in them dissipated under my fingers and his breathing deepened.

I slowly dragged my palms over his butt cheeks, which were tight. I asked Kevin to breathe in and bring his attention to my hands. He inhaled deeply and his hips loosened as he exhaled.

I worked my way up until I reached the crown of his head.

Kevin's eyes were closed and each breath he took was so deep that I thought he might have fallen asleep.

"Kevin?" I said softly.

He started.

"How are you doing?"

"I was dozing off. This is so relaxing."

"Good. I'm glad you're relaxed. I'm going to work my way down your body again."

I gradually moved from Kevin's head to his toes.

Then I asked him to take a deep breath and, when he was ready, to roll over onto his back.

His penis stood almost straight up, and it remained that way for the whole time I touched the front of his body.

That Kevin had no problem maintaining an erection with me, especially in our first session, made me more curious about the dynamic between him and Diane. As we continued to see each other, a pattern emerged. He would get an erection almost as soon as we got undressed, and while it might wane, it never totally left.

When we did the Sexological in our fourth session, Kevin remained hard throughout. It was in the feedback period after I had stimulated him with my mouth and hand when the mystery of why he could sustain an erection with me, but not with Diane was solved, and it provided yet another reminder of the importance of basic communication.

I asked Kevin the usual questions about what he liked best.

"Definitely when you went down on me. I'd forgotten how much I liked that."

I was surprised by his answer because I remembered him saying that he and Diane had oral sex and that it was then when he typically lost his erection.

"Does Diane not like to give you blow jobs?"

"She does it, but it hurts me."

"What about it hurts?"

"She uses her teeth and they scrape against my penis."

"Have you talked to her about this?"

"No, I can't."

"Why not?"

"I don't want to hurt her feelings."

"Kevin, you can tell her about this without hurting her feelings. You'd want her to tell you if you were doing something that hurt, right?"

"Yeah, but . . . what if she thinks I'm criticizing her?"

"Well, I can't promise how she'll react, but there are communication techniques that can help limit the chances that she'll take this as a personal criticism."

I asked Kevin if Diane was open to talking about sex.

"Yeah. She really wants to understand what's stopping us from having it. She jokes about sex a lot, and she's not shy in bed. She was happy when I told her I was coming here because she wants to, well, get laid."

"That's a great starting point."

I sat down next to Kevin on the bed and shared some of the best communication techniques I know.

"Start by explaining that you want to talk about this because you love her and find her attractive and you want your sex life to be mutually satisfying. If you help her to see the ultimate purpose of the discussion, she's more likely to want to participate in it."

Kevin listened attentively.

"Use 'I' statements. No accusing or scolding. You might say something like, 'I really love when you go down on me, but when you press down with your teeth I feel some pain and it diminishes my hard-on."

"What if she gets embarrassed?"

"Remind her that you want to know if you're doing something that doesn't feel good to her. Give her the same opportunity she's giving you."

"I wonder if I am doing something she doesn't like," Kevin said.

"Talking honestly and openly with each other is the only way to find out. Let Diane know that you want the lines of communication to stay open. Your likes and dislikes may change and hers might too. You have to be able to talk to each other about that as you grow and age together."

For the first time Kevin blushed and he averted his eyes from me. He looked embarrassed.

"How are you feeling?"

"Well, a little silly to tell you the truth."

When I asked him why, he said it was because the solution to his problem had been there all along, and now it seemed so simple.

"It may look simple, but remember, few of us are taught how to communicate about sex."

"I just . . . just assumed we couldn't talk about that for some reason."

"You just needed the encouragement and reminder that you can. There's nothing magical here. These are simple skills that you can learn. Are you going to try to talk to Diane today?"

"I don't know. It seems like it should be easy, but I get scared when I think of telling her about this."

Kevin and I role-played some possible scenarios that might unfold between them. A quick study, he became more and more adept at communicating his concern without criticism as we practiced.

Kevin and I saw each other for two more sessions. At our last one he told me he had finally gotten up the nerve to talk to Diane.

"She was so happy that I told her. She said she wished she had known sooner," he said cheerfully.

For the first time in months, they had had intercourse.

I was happy that Kevin had finally been able to have sex with Diane again, but I was happier that he had opened the communication between them and laid the groundwork for an ongoing fulfilling sex life. He had learned one of the essential secrets of all great lovers.

16.

isn't that your daughter?

The backlash was on. In 1986, we were in the thick of Ronald Reagan's second term and the United States was moving ever more rightward. The gains of the Sexual Revolution and other social movements were imperiled by an alignment of traditional conservative forces and the Religious Right. It seemed as though we were turning the clock back to a time when sexuality was demonized and sexual concerns were suppressed.

Reagan remained mum about AIDS until 1987, after thousands had already been felled by it. The Moral Majority and other right-wing activists appropriated the disease as a political weapon and took aim at the gay community, one of their favorite scapegoats. Unalloyed victim blaming and withering condemnation spewed from the grass-roots bullhorns to the fundamentalist pulpits to the national media channels open to government officials. "The poor homosexuals—they have declared war upon nature, and now nature is extracting an awful retribution," Pat Buchanan, Reagan's communications director, inveighed in *The New York Post* in 1986. The time was ripe for an attack on reproductive rights, sexual minorities, and women; the march backward had begun.

It was naïve, but I sometimes thought if these hateful bullies would simply listen to one of the legion of AIDS patients who they summarily damned they might see that they were talking about real human beings and not a mass of faceless demons. If they could listen to my dear friend Steven Brown, for example, they might change their point of view.

By the early '80s, Steven and I had become fixtures on the training staff at San Francisco Sex Information. We met twice a year to train new crops of volunteers who kept the organization thriving.

In the winter of 1986, we prepared a class of fifty people. On the first day of training, Steven, myself, and other teachers traded off addressing the group, answering questions, and running through dozens of hypothetical scenarios they might encounter as phone volunteers.

When our lunch break rolled around, an unannounced rain crashed down on the city, and neither Steven nor I had an umbrella. We pulled our coats over our heads and headed to a Chinese place just a couple of blocks from the SFSI training site. About halfway there we started running, and by the time we swung the door open to the warm restaurant we were both out of breath and laughing like school kids.

We wedged ourselves into a red vinyl booth, and the waiter placed a steaming pot of tea between us. Steven poured a cup for me and then one for himself. I wrapped my fingers tightly around the ceramic mug to warm my hands. The sizzling noise of stir-frying came from the kitchen and mingled with the savory smells of pepper and garlic. I realized I was famished. We ordered and sipped our tea while we waited for lunch.

"Good group this time around," I said.

"Yeah, every year they seem to arrive better educated."

"Remember when we started in the seventies? How little most of us knew?"

Steven said nothing. He turned his cup around with his fingertips and fiddled with his silverware. Then he looked me in the eyes.

"Cheryl, I have to tell you something."

His mood had turned serious and I felt a sudden dread.

"I got tested," he said.

Oh no, I thought.

Our egg rolls arrived and we both looked at them and then at each other.

"I'm HIV positive."

"Oh, Steven . . . " I said, and felt my stomach drop.

How much longer will he live? It was an eerie thought. What he told me was that he was HIV positive. What I heard was that he would be dead soon. I imagined his handsome face drawn and sallow.

"Steven, I . . . "

"Cheryl, it's okay. The truth is, I wasn't shocked to get the news."

Steven had enjoyed a lot of partners. Maybe I shouldn't have been shocked either, but I just sat there unable to speak.

"I'm learning everything I can about how to stay healthy. I'm going to fight this for as long as I can, and I'm not alone," he said.

I squeezed Steven's hand. "No, you're not. Not at all."

When we returned to the training that afternoon, I marveled at how Steven dove back into his work without hesitation. I never would have guessed that anything was wrong as he cracked jokes and addressed the class in his usual animated and dynamic style. Steven was up against a pitiless disease, but he was facing it with the same positive, take-charge spirit that made me and so many others fall in love with him.

True to his word, Steven became a lay expert on HIV and AIDS. He educated himself and his friends on the best self-care after diagnosis. Before his diagnosis, Steven frequented the bathhouses, where gay men met to engage in casual sex. What was left of the bathhouse scene now included volunteer safer sex patrols and he signed on to be part of them. He became part of a crew that monitored the Sutro bathhouse to ensure that everyone engaged in safer play. In addition to taking a drug cocktail, he maintained a healthy lifestyle and a positive attitude. Steven continued to work as a surrogate, and he was scrupulous about telling all clients upfront about his condition and using condoms and other safer sex measures.

⟡

Most days it felt like I helplessly watched as the hard-won triumphs of the '60s and '70s became the targets of this new era. The only thing I could do was talk—publicly. I could at least try to present my perspective, one that was being drowned out by the shrill cries of the revived and energized Puritans and professional finger-waggers. I had been interviewed for local TV and print media in the past. I wanted people to understand what surrogates do, but I also wanted to do my small part in demystifying and destigmatizing sex by making it part of the public discussion. That took on a renewed importance now.

It wasn't uncommon for Steven and I to do media together. "The Steven and Cheryl Show," as we dubbed ourselves, began in the mid-'80s when we appeared on a local Bay Area program called *People Are Talking*. Often producers who found one of us would ask if we could refer them to other surrogates. Some media handled our work thoughtfully; others played up the most sensational aspects. It was always a gamble, and I wasn't sure how to best hedge my bets. Was it worth having a sensational piece for the larger mission of changing the public discussion, or did it just feed into all the same old stale, misleading narratives and myths?

The Steven and Cheryl Show got its national TV break when *Larry King Live* booked us for an interview in 1989. This was one of the first national programs to take on surrogacy work and I was nervous. Larry King was a TV legend, and what if my parents stumbled on it? They had only a vague idea of what I did for a living, and the last thing they would do was press for more details. They knew it involved sex and sexuality, so it couldn't be good.

The producers of the show arranged for us to film in a Los Angeles studio so we didn't have to fly to DC where the program was based. Unlike some other shows I had done, I wasn't expected to show up "camera ready." As soon as we arrived at the studio, Steven and I were whisked off to makeup artists. When I was done I had so much makeup on that I feared I looked clownish. "Don't worry, you'll look great onscreen," the makeup artist assured me. I took another look in the mirror and hoped she was right. I felt and looked like I had on a mask.

An assistant then led me on to a soundstage where Steven was waiting for me. It had been close to two years since his diagnosis and he still looked handsome and fit. The doctors marveled at how well Steven was doing, and I was eternally grateful for it.

"Hey, Bruce Willis was the last person to sit in this seat," a giddy Steven said to me.

"Really? Who sat here last?" I asked one of the crew members, pointing at my chair.

"Zsa Zsa Gabor," he answered.

"Wow, Zsa Zsa's was the last butt to touch this seat. How about that?" I said to Steven.

"Bruce, Zsa Zsa, Steven, and Cheryl. It was meant to be," he said.

We both laughed until a sound engineer clipped microphones on us.

There were three cameras on us, and the producer explained that a red light would indicate which one was taping. We should look into the active camera throughout the show. I took some deep breaths and told myself to stay calm and confident. Then Larry appeared on a monitor, and within minutes we were live on the air. King asked reasonable questions and he allowed us to answer them fully. Only one caller was overtly hostile. When it was over, Steven and I both felt like we had been given a fair opportunity to explain what we do and why it matters.

When I got home I watched the video that Michael made of the show. The makeup artist was right! For once, I looked good on TV.

A few days later I called home to check in on my parents. Exactly what I had feared had happened. My father's friend had recognized me and called him. "Bob," he said, "isn't that your daughter on *Larry King Live?*" Here we go, I thought when my father told me he had watched the interview. To my surprise he simply said, "So that's what you do." "Yes, Dad. I educate people about sexuality and help them feel more comfortable with it," I answered.

I could account for my father's unexpectedly easy response in a few ways. To be sure, he had mellowed with age, but I sensed there was something deeper at play. I think my dad had decided that he wanted a relationship with me and that meant he had to accept me for who I was. The father I grew up with would have been mortified by the disclosure I had made on national TV. While I didn't ask him to confirm it, I also thought that he may have even seen the value in what I do. When King had asked me how I help people as a surrogate, I responded that few of us grow up with any credible sex education. Our ideas about what our sex lives should be come from conversations with our friends, movies, books, and pornography—all notoriously unreliable sources. With that kind of misinformation, it's no wonder so many people are confused and distressed. I explained that a big part of my work is to educate people so that they have more realistic expectations of themselves and others. My father's generation, those who came of age in the '30s, and mine in the '50s, lacked any reliable sex education. We both had grown up in a time when talking about sex was taboo. I was trying to share what I had learned so that later generations wouldn't come of sexual age in an information vacuum. Maybe he actually thought that was worthwhile. At any rate, he ended the conversation with, "Let us know the next time you're on TV."

My mother stayed tight-lipped until my next visit, which came about four months later. Several years earlier, Mom and Dad had moved from Massachusetts to New Hampshire. When I arrived in early summer it was so hot that I spent most of the time indoors, where the temperature was made arctic by the air conditioner squeezed into the living room window. I had hoped my mother would bring up the show, but by the third day of my visit I recognized that if I wanted to discuss it I would have to make the first move. I was proud of how I had handled myself in the interview, and I thought Steven and I offered a realistic depiction of surrogacy work. As my mother watched the news one evening, I sat down next to her on the couch. I asked her if she had seen *Larry King* along with Dad, even though I was almost certain she had. She nodded and sat up a little straighter. I thought of just dropping it, but I pushed ahead. I was going to explain my work to my mother. If I was prepared to reveal and defend my profession before the American public, I could do it in front of my mother.

"I'm glad you saw it," I said, wagering, perhaps unrealistically, that our talk would go well.

Mom said nothing.

"I thought I did a good job of explaining my work."

I wanted my mother to agree with me, or disagree, or tell me to shut up, or just say something. Instead she just stared at me, her face resolutely neutral.

"I'm trying to help people feel less ashamed and confused about sexuality. We don't come from a culture that opens up comfortably about it. We barely talk about it, and parents aren't given any education about how to talk to their kids. There's nothing I like more than helping people feel more comfortable with their sexuality, and have more information than I did."

I stopped there because I didn't want it to seem like I was accusing her. I was tired of fighting with my mother.

"You don't have to talk about that stuff. It just happens naturally," she said.

She'd finally said something. It was wrong, but she had piped up and at least acknowledged me.

"No, Mom, it doesn't. Our brains are too complex for it just to happen naturally. We live in a culture that's negative about sexuality. We don't approach it from an informed perspective, and we're given constant mixed messages about it. Sex may be natural, but it doesn't happen naturally."

I looked at my mother, trying to gauge whether any of what I was saying was getting through to her, but she maintained an expressionless face. We sat there and looked at each other for a few seconds. Although my mother was pretty icy, I had to acknowledge that she wasn't screaming at me or accusing me of scandalous behavior.

"Do you remember when I told Larry King that I work with disabled people? Well, that's one of the most rewarding parts of my job, and I'm able to work with them as well as I do because of you."

"Me?"

"Yes, you. Do you remember Greta next door?"

Greta was the developmentally disabled girl whom my mother always treated with such dignity and respect. Once I came home and found the then twelve-year-old Greta sitting on our back steps crying. Blood trickled down her legs in two thin red stripes. My mother took Greta in, helped her bathe, and gave her a sanitary napkin. She sat her down at our kitchen table and made her a cup of tea, all the while talking to her in a reassuring but not patronizing voice. There was a boy who had a facial deformity who worked at the bus station that we would sometimes use. My mother always said hello and smiled at him just as she would anyone else.

"The way you treated them taught me a lesson about respecting everyone. It also taught me to look beyond what you see on the outside. I think about that a lot when I work with disabled people."

My mother and I stared at each other. I wasn't going to say anything. She would have to break the silence.

"I don't know where you come from. You're like nobody else in this family," she said.

At least now she was calling me different. In the past she had called me so much worse. Maybe this wasn't a warm and fuzzy moment, but it was progress.

I still grappled with which kind of media to engage with and which outlets to avoid. This was the beginning of the "trash TV" explosion, and a number of daytime talk shows jockeyed to be the most shocking, most titillating hour of the day. A year earlier Geraldo Rivera had waded into the fray with *Geraldo*. I had watched the show a few times and I knew that it was unabashedly sensationalistic, and that's what I had to consider when they called several months after my *Larry King Live* appearance.

Marty Klein, a local therapist who I knew from SFSI and other organizations, had just published *Your Sexual Secrets: When to Keep Them, When and How to Tell*, and Geraldo was putting together a show based on this theme. Years ago I had confessed what I thought was a secret to Michael: that I sometimes masturbated to achieve orgasm if sex with him didn't bring me to climax. I thought I was sparing his feelings and protecting his ego by waiting until he fell asleep before starting. When I told him about it, he was unfazed. In fact, he said it wasn't much of a secret at all because he wasn't always asleep when I thought he was. I had told Marty about this, and when the Geraldo producer asked if he knew a couple who had faced a secret, he sent him to me.

I knew that I couldn't expect an in-depth discussion or debate on the show, but still, it was a chance to talk openly about sex in a national forum. I thought about Brian, my client whose wife left him for masturbating. If we could talk openly about this and other sexual practices, maybe we could reduce the suffering of people like Brian, not to mention his wife. So, even though I knew I wasn't going to receive the most sensitive treatment, I went to New York with Michael to tape the episode. Remembering Dad's request, I let my parents know that I was going to be interviewed on TV again.

Along with Marty Klein, Michael, and myself, the panel included a sex worker whose primary clientele were people with infantilism, a client of hers who secretly engaged in it, and a women who kept her exhibitionism under wraps.

To no one's great surprise, the panel was treated as a freak show, a menagerie of oddballs on display for the amusement of the general public. The guest with infantilism, a little-understood condition in which people become aroused by being treated like babies, sat behind a screen and talked about how he liked to be bottle-fed and wear diapers. The exhibitionist revealed that she liked to have sex in phone booths and other public places. I must have seemed downright dull compared to them. They were on the fringes of human sexuality. I was just Cheryl Cohen, Secret Masturbator, or at least that's how the caption under my face identified me to the viewing audience. Decades after I had masturbated on the sly because of guilt and shame, I had come out to the world as a secret masturbator. I had to admit I was a little amused by it. What would the nuns at St. Mary's say? What would the priests say? What would my family say? The answer to that last question came soon enough.

"Burn it." That was my beloved grandmother's response when my cousin Jean showed her the VHS tape she had made of it. I talked to my cousin over the phone about a week after the show aired, and we laughed about Nanna Fournier's response, but the tone got much more sober when it came to my parents. They had not said a word to anyone about the show and no one dared to ask. I was scheduled to visit them back East in a few months. They would either break their silence or they wouldn't, and I wasn't sure which worried me more.

Most in my crowd of friends and acquaintances responded to the show in a uniformly dispassionate way. If they had one complaint it was that it was a shame that an opportunity to have a national conversation about taboo subjects was reduced to an exercise in voyeurism. I decided that I would avoid outlets that I thought would sensationalize without making at least a token effort at serious discussion and education.

When I talked to my mother on the phone, I could hear the anger in her voice. If I thought we had made a modicum of progress when we talked about the Larry King interview, I now suspected that we were about to take a leap backward.

In a rare move, Michael decided to join me for the trip back East. As it neared, we needed to pick up a few travel items, and the Saturday before we were due to leave we got in the car and drove around Berkeley buying supplies. As we rolled up to a stop sign, a police car came up next to my side of the car and the driver beeped the horn. "What do they want? We haven't done anything," I said to Michael. The cop behind the wheel motioned for me to roll down the window. My stomach tightened as I cranked it down about halfway. There were two officers in the car and they were both smiling. "Hey, weren't you guys on *Geraldo?*" the driver asked. "Good work," they both said, and gave us a thumbs-up. Michael and I breathed a sigh of relief. Only in Berkeley. I loved living in the land where cops would applaud you for revealing a sexual secret on national TV, and where few people failed to understand my mission even if they thought doing the show didn't exactly further it.

When Michael and I arrived at my parents' house, I was reminded of just how much of a bubble good-old Berkeley is. My mother's response was frosty from the outset. She couldn't even muster a smile when we walked through the door. It was a shame. She was getting old. She had fine lines etched around her mouth and across her forehead. Would we make peace before it was too late? Luckily, Michael and I arrived at night so we excused ourselves and headed off to bed.

At breakfast the next morning I tried to steer the conversation toward topics I knew would please my parents. I talked about Jessica and Eric and how well they were doing. Michael stuck to talk about the weather. We polished off our eggs and toast quickly, and as soon as we were done we went our separate ways. Michael and I dashed out for a walk in the beautiful New England fall. The oak and maple trees looked like they were on fire with their dazzling array of yellow and orange and red. We walked hand in hand to the town center.

"Well, this has been fun," Michael said sarcastically.

"I know. It's the show. I know this is about *Geraldo,*" I said.

It had been around four or five months since the show had aired, and my mother's anger hadn't waned.

"I'm going to confront her about it when we get back. I'm sick of walking around on pins and needles. If she's going to freak out, let's get it over with."

"Okay, but it's probably best if I stay clear," Michael replied.

"Of course it is."

The crisp fall air was laced with the scent of burning firewood. It smelled comforting and homey. I only wished I was heading back to another home.

I could hear the sound of the TV when we walked through the door. I peeked into the living room and saw Mom sitting on the couch. My father was gone, probably running errands. Michael kissed me and headed to the kitchen.

I lowered the volume on the TV and sat next to my mother on the couch that was covered in brown upholstery.

"Mom, I know you saw the show and you're angry," I said.

She glared at me.

"I did it because I want people to stop being ashamed of things they shouldn't be ashamed of."

My mother flushed.

"It is shameful. It's sickening how you behave!" she screamed.

Now I was irate, not just at her but at myself. My mother had once again managed to infuriate me and I was frustrated with myself for allowing her to get me angry.

"No, Mom, it's not. I haven't done anything wrong and you need to understand that. What's sick is pretending that there's something wrong with sex."

I stood up and started pacing across a rug that lay on the floor in front of the couch.

"This is his fault. I don't know why you let Michael control you like this."

"What are you talking about?"

"I know you only did that because he wanted you to."

Now not only was I furious, but insulted and hurt. Did she think I was just Michael's pawn? Was I just a fool who couldn't think for myself?

"You're wrong. If you knew me at all you'd know that!"

I stomped out of the living room.

"Let's get out of here!" I shouted to Michael.

We threw our clothes into a suitcase, slammed it shut, and left for the nearest motel.

The only thing that stopped Michael and me from getting on the next plane to California was that I planned to see Nanna Fournier the next day. She was now eighty-seven years old. Her hair was peppered with grey and she walked with a limp from the arthritis that had overrun her body, but she was still as sharp-witted as ever. Her joie de vivre had carried her intact through a life with its share of hardships.

"Is that you?" Nanna called when I knocked on the door of her apartment in Salem. "It's me," I answered. She opened the door and flung her arms open wide. "Cheryl!" she cried. "Nanna!" I yelled back, and planted a big kiss on her lovely face. We hugged each other and then Nanna leaned on me for support as we walked to the kitchen. She took a pound cake out of the refrigerator and put the kettle on for tea.

We gossiped about family members and joked about her losing the figure that she used to love to dress up in the latest fashions. Even still, she looked more stylish than most women her age. She continued to wear lipstick and had taken to wearing a wig. It was as if I had never left. She told me, once again, the story about my sweet but somewhat dopey uncle whom she watched one summer afternoon as he sat in an maple tree sawing away on an overgrown limb. He forgot that he sat on the very arm he was cutting off until he crashed to the ground with it. It never got old, especially the way Nanna Fournier told it.

If I had never mentioned the *Geraldo* appearance, I know Nanna wouldn't have broached it. I wanted to talk about it, though, because I wanted her to know that I cared about her opinion and I wanted a chance to explain myself to her.

I carved a second slice of cake and looked at my grandmother squarely.

"Nanna, I know you saw the TV show I was on."

"Cheryl, I couldn't believe it," she said.

"Why?"

"Why? Because of what you talked about. That's personal. You don't talk about those things in public."

"No, Nanna. We need to talk about it. We have to stop being ashamed of sexuality and we have to stop keeping it a secret."

Nanna took a bite of her cake and looked at me with a little smile.

"You're not mad, are you?" I asked.

"At you? I can't be. Nothing you do could make me angry. If you were lying in a gutter I'd get in there and lie beside you," she said.

My heart felt like it was going to burst. When I was a kid I thought that if my grandmother knew how I sinned she would turn against me. I had no idea, when I was a secret masturbator, that her love was this unconditional.

17.

the fantasy: derek

"**H**e's different than other clients I've referred to you," Samantha said. We were in her office on a late afternoon in the winter of 1990. Samantha and I had worked together several times over the past few years, and as I sat across from her I wondered what could be so unusual about this potential client.

"How so?"

"He's struggling with an obsessive fantasy that's causing real problems in his marriage and his life."

"What kind of fantasy?"

"It stems from an experience he had as a kid. When he was around eight, his babysitter was a neighborhood girl of around twelve or thirteen. She used to tie him to a tree in the backyard and then slap him or dance around taunting him."

"I think I know where this is going," I said.

Samantha smiled.

It's not unusual for erotic preferences to be shaped by childhood experiences, and I had a feeling that this was the case with Derek, the client Samantha was describing.

"He gets turned on by the thought of being restrained. He's told his wife about it and she's called him 'sick.' She won't consider acting it out with him, and right now it's what excites him the most."

"Is he able to have sex with his wife at all?"

"Yes, but he feels like he's mostly doing it to pleasure her. The whole time he fantasizes about being tied up and then he feels guilty. I think if he could act out his fantasy it might help him break the obsession with it."

This wasn't what I normally did as a surrogate, and it would mean deviating from protocol. I wasn't completely comfortable with this, but I also trusted Samantha's instincts and I knew I would be safe with Derek.

Samantha and I talked more about what my work with him would entail. I could go through the regular exercises, but our primary focus would be on acting out the fantasy in the hopes that it would loosen his obsession with it. I was unsure, not only because it was so outside the bounds of what I typically do, but also because my tastes are pretty "vanilla" when it comes to sex, and I didn't relish the idea of getting someone off by taunting him.

When I left Samantha's office that day, she told me she would pass on my contact information to him. The next day he called to make an appointment.

Derek was in his mid-forties. He was tall, with a strong build and brown hair. That he desperately wanted to stay with his wife, with whom he had three children, came through almost immediately in our first conversation.

"I don't want to lose my wife, especially not over this," he said.

I asked Derek to talk a little about the discussion he had had with his wife, Melanie, about his fantasy.

"She likes sex and she initiates it a lot, but the idea of, well, what

I'm into—it really turns her off. She says she can't humiliate someone she loves. Before I started seeing Samantha we got into a big fight about it."

"Is that why you went to therapy in the first place?"

"Yeah, it was what she said about my fantasies that made me go."

I asked Derek to describe their fight.

"She wanted to have sex and I wasn't really interested. I mean, I can't get turned on unless I fantasize about being tied up, and I was trying not to do that. I was trying to force the fantasy out of my mind and to get turned on by her kissing me, but she could tell that I wasn't into it."

Derek paused and looked off to the side.

"She got really mad, and she said I should just go get a mistress who would tie me up or find someone who I could pay for it. I told her I didn't want that and that I loved her. She started yelling at me and said I was sick. After she calmed down she apologized and said she didn't mean it, but I guess I wonder if she's right."

Derek stared at me with a look that expressed something between expectation and desperation. He wanted to hear that he wasn't "sick."

"Sexuality is very complex and sometimes childhood experiences can determine what we desire in later life," I said.

Since Derek wasn't feeling satisfied with his wife, I wondered if he was engaging in other activities. When I asked him about this, he squeezed his hands on the armrests of the chair and nodded.

"What kinds of things do you do?"

Derek closed his eyes and took a deep breath.

Then he told me that when his wife and children were gone he broke out a box that he had hidden in the attic. It held a corset and a pair of support hose that were the smallest size he could fit in to. Dressing up in these items simulated the feeling he'd had as a child when his babysitter tied him up. He could feel his penis growing against the pressure of the constricting hose, and just before he felt he was going to ejaculate, he would rip them off. Sometimes he masturbated himself, but other times he came without any direct stimulation.

"I feel like I've built up this parallel life around my fantasy, and I have so many secrets because of it. Once when my wife and kids went away to her parents' house for the weekend, I spent the whole time in the garage working on a . . . a . . . device."

"A device?" I asked.

"Yeah, I built it a while ago. It's been hidden in my garage for a long time."

"What does it do?"

"It's something I could be tied to. I also have rope."

"Have you used it before?"

"No, but . . . I'm hoping we can use it together."

Derek asked if he could bring it to our next session. I was a little apprehensive, but I agreed to take a look at it.

Derek and I talked for a little while longer. He described his fantasy in great detail. He even had a script he had written that spelled out what each player would say and do, and he asked if he could show it to me.

He wanted me to dance around him after I tied him up and then gently touch his penis, but not jerk him off or bring him to orgasm. He also said he wanted to have intercourse afterward. By the time he was done, I had a vivid picture of what he was hoping to experience. He left the script with me so I could review it before our next meeting. We decided we would see each other once a month for the next five months.

⌒

When I opened the door to let Derek in for our second session, I was greeted by a contraption that was about six-foot tall and hidden beneath a black tarp. I could see two points sticking up about three feet apart from each other. He lifted it with both hands and carried it into my office.

"I brought it," he said.

"I see."

We talked for a little while. In the last month, Derek's fantasy had continued to intrude into his life. He found himself wondering if attractive women he passed on the street would be willing to tie him up. Melanie was getting frustrated with his lack of progress. He did his best to feign interest in sex with her, but he couldn't ejaculate unless he thought of himself being restrained. He didn't tell her, but he had been looking forward to today's session ever since he'd left our first one.

"Are you ready to head to the bedroom?" I asked Derek.

He lifted up the mysterious device with both hands and followed me down the hall to the bedroom. He had to turn sideways to comfortably fit it through the door.

Before I asked Derek to disrobe, I asked him to remove the tarp that covered his invention. He pulled it off, and there it was. It was beautifully constructed out of what looked like cedar. It had two tall posts that were held together by a latticework. The bottom of the posts flared out and had rubber tips fitted to them to ensure that they wouldn't slip. Along the two legs were large metal loops, like those that would go with a hook-and-eye closure. Derek unzipped the gym bag he had brought with him and lifted out a coil of white rope. He showed me how the rope would weave through the metal loops.

"You've obviously put a lot of thought and hard work into this," I said.

"Yeah, it's something I've thought about for years."

We both undressed and went through a round of Spoon Breathing. I taught him a few relaxation techniques. Then, when I normally would have asked if he was ready to begin Sensual Touch, I asked if Derek was ready to act out the fantasy he had dreamed of for decades.

He stood up and shook out his arms.

"I can hardly believe this is happening," he said.

It's new for me too, I thought.

My apprehension was starting to slip away a little. I had reread the script that morning and I was relieved that I could take my lead from

it. Taunting someone wasn't part of my professional or personal repertoire. I had friends who liked this kind of play, but it just wasn't for
me. I thought back to the script and silently thanked Derek for being
so well prepared.

Derek walked over to the device, pressed his back up against the latticework, which I could now see extended from the backs of his calves
to just above his shoulder blades. I picked up the rope and threaded
it through the bottom left loop. Derek guided me through making a
square knot to ensure that it would be firmly anchored to the frame.
I walked to the right and threaded it through the corresponding loop,
then I went up through the second set of loops, and the third, and
the fourth, until the rope made a zigzag pattern all along the front of
Derek's body. "Tighter," Derek said when I pulled the rope through
the last loop and crossed it over to make a knot. I tugged a little harder
and he smiled. "That's it," he said.

Derek was now wedged between the lattice and the rope. I asked
him if he was ready to take the next step. His breath picked up and his
face and body were flushed.

"Uh-huh," he said, nearly breathless.

I stood about three feet away from him and started circling around
him.

"Does that feel good?" I asked. "I hope so because I'm going to
leave you there for days."

With each revolution I got a little closer until I was close enough to
touch him if I stretched out my arm.

I lightly crossed his chest with my fingers and wiggled them as I
moved along his warm skin. Derek watched me as I pranced around
nude. For a few seconds I felt self-conscious and awkward. To pull
myself back into the moment I thought about the long nights with
Bob when we spent hours tasting and touching, caressing and masturbating each other. We had intercourse sometimes three or four times
in one night, and as I recalled this I started to feel more aroused and
my discomfort faded.

I tweaked Derek's nipples, soft at first and then a little harder.

"Oooh, what's going on down here?" I said looking at his hardening penis.

Derek let out a few little squeals.

Then I backed off and started orbiting around him again.

"Do you want to kiss me?"

Derek nodded his head.

I brought my lips within a hair of his and then pulled back.

"You'll have to be quicker than that," I said.

Derek panted. His lips were engorged and had turned a bright cherry red.

I licked around his nipples and then moved my tongue up his chest and throat.

"What's this?" I asked as I wiped pre-come off the tip of his penis.

I smeared it on his lips.

"Do you like that?"

Derek licked his lips.

I rubbed my breasts on his abdomen.

"Am I exciting you?"

He tried to maneuver his hands to his penis, but he was too tightly bound.

"What's that you're trying to do?" I asked.

I circled around him a few times.

"If I didn't know better, I'd think you wanted to touch your cock."

I traced around his penis with my index finger.

"Oh, aaahhhh," Derek said.

"Ready?" I asked.

He nodded, and I undid the rope at the top. I pulled it quickly through the first loop and then worked my way down to the last one until it fell on the ground with a soft thud.

He grabbed my shoulders and kissed me while we walked to the bed. I quickly unrolled a condom onto his penis and we lay down next to each other. Soon he was on top of me and we were having intercourse. After he came, he rolled over next to me and panted, "Thank you, thank you, thank you."

I put my arm around Derek and led him in some deep breathing. This was an important moment for him, and I wanted to be as supportive as I could. Our work together was less of a shared experience than with most of my clients, and it was also simpler and more straightforward. We weren't exploring and trading feedback. We were together solely to bring Derek's fantasy to life, so that it might loosen its grip on him.

In each of our four remaining sessions Derek and I acted out his fantasy. I also did some of the standard surrogacy exercises with him. Despite the alternative focus of our work together, I still thought it might help Derek discover and cultivate other sources of arousal. I grew more at ease with my role as midwife to Derek's fantasy, especially when I started to see a change in him.

Samantha and I were curious if her theory would prove right. Would finally living out his fantasy help Derek to become less obsessed with it? It was in the fourth session that he first reported to me that his fixation with being tied up was fading, and he didn't get as aroused as quickly as he did in our earlier visits. The idea of being restrained still excited him, but it wasn't intruding into his life as much, and he was able to enjoy sex with Melanie more. When I spoke with Samantha after my last session with Derek she reported that he and Melanie has started to find mutual sources of arousal, and while he still indulged in his fantasy, it no longer had a monopoly on his desire.

Working with Derek reminded me of the need for flexibility in the surrogacy process. Sexuality is complicated and some clients benefit from stepping outside of the protocol. I had been a surrogate for close to two decades when I saw him and I never imagined I would work with a client in this way. That Derek responded so well reminded me of the value of hands-on work, even when it takes a form that stretches beyond the usual parameters. That traditional therapy and surrogacy can be a powerful combination was underscored for me once again.

18.

monsieur reaper

....

Michael's two children with Meg spent a few weeks in Northern California with us every summer. They were delightful kids who had bonded with Jessica and Eric, and had stolen my heart. At forty-eight, having two wonderful younger kids who I didn't have to provide for was a joy. In addition to his daughter, Michael now had a second son. By the late '80s they were both old enough to travel without Meg, and when summer arrived they came with us to Berkeley Tuolumne Camp near Yosemite, where we took long hikes, went swimming, and did other fun activities as an unconventional family.

Michael still made regular visits to see the kids in the Pacific Northwest, but when the oldest was four-and-a-half, he asked if she could come visit and I couldn't refuse. No matter how angry I was at Michael, I couldn't justify denying his daughter a chance to see her father and become a greater part of his everyday life, even if it was only a few times a year. Later his son began making the trips too. I soon went from allowing the visits to looking forward to them.

My kids also bonded with their half-siblings. Telling them that their father had made a baby with another woman wasn't easy. After the birth of Michael's daughter, we sat them down one evening and I explained that they now had a little sister. Their first concern was for me. I admitted that I wasn't happy with their father, who was uncharacteristically silent at this family meeting. I stressed that the new baby deserved to be loved. I felt no resentment toward her, and I hoped that they didn't either. When the second child came along, their concern, again, was primarily for me. Jessica and Eric had been raised in an unconventional household, so this news probably wasn't as shocking to them as it might have been to other kids. They had met Meg and had even traveled with Michael a few times to visit her.

As far as I knew, Meg was happy to have a part-time husband and father for her kids, or at least that's what I told myself. Michael never said anything to the contrary, but then Michael knew better than to raise the subject of Meg with me. It was just one of the many topics that could spark an argument.

For virtually all of our marriage I had harbored a jumble of feelings toward Michael. I showered him with adoration and affection, while only occasionally giving voice to the anger and resentment that quietly brewed within me. It had to be like that. I loved Michael so deeply and I was so grateful that he was my husband that I couldn't risk alienating him. That changed, however, when he had his second family. The anger hardened into a contempt I had difficulty concealing. I could feel myself turning bitter, nursing a rage that could poison not just my marriage, but my life. The slightest jolt could release a flood of the vitriol that simmered below the surface.

In truth, this wasn't just about Michael. Without a doubt, I had changed too. A couple of years shy of fifty, I had more confidence and self-esteem than I had ever had in my life. I deserved better than the indignities Michael had foisted on me. His reckless, insensitive behavior and my hard-won confidence combined to give me a new perspective on Michael. Having a loving, supportive partner in Bob also boosted my sense of self-worth. He loved me unconditionally and it changed how I saw myself.

I was sick of never feeling good enough for Michael and tired of fighting with him, and for him. Life without him no longer seemed like a death sentence. In fact, I could imagine getting along just fine without him as my husband. My confidence may have come late, but there was no mistaking that it had arrived. Jessica was now twenty-seven and Eric twenty-four. They were busily creating their own lives, and they could continue their relationship with their father without me staying married to him.

I knew the process of separating from him would be difficult. Michael, after all, was deeply enmeshed in my life. I had spent most of my life with him. I wasn't even sure I would be able to look at him and tell him it was over. When I thought about it, I got teary. Our relationship was on life support, but that didn't mean pulling the plug would be easy.

In 1992, Michael and I went to Boston to attend my thirtieth high school reunion. In public, Michael donned the charming persona I had seen him cultivate over the years. He smiled and looked into my eyes as we danced together. Anyone watching would have thought our marriage was as solid, as permanent as the nearby Berkshire Mountains. If only they had seen us on the plane, or a few days earlier when Michael acted like talking to me was a favor. I suspected his coldness had something to do with Andrea, his new girlfriend.

Michael met Andrea at SFSI, the same place he'd met Meg. The first time I saw them talking together I knew they were sleeping together, and when I confronted him he didn't bother to deny it. So much for my Ahwahnee declaration that Meg would be the only woman he saw outside of me. With Andrea and Meg he now had two women on the side—that I knew of. To discover that he had betrayed me once again hurt, but it was no surprise. That he didn't feel the need to deny it, however, was a relief because it spared me the struggle of teasing it out of him, and it was yet another signal that the marriage was nothing more than a shell.

On the flight back to Berkeley, Michael barely spoke to me. When I asked him to lift my bag into the overhead compartment he shot me a sour look and snatched it out of my hand. I don't think more than ten words were exchanged on the entire trip home. By the time we settled in to bed I was fuming.

"What's the problem, Michael?" I demanded.

"Nothing."

"Oh, come on. You've been ignoring me since we left for Boston."

Michael paused for a few seconds, as though he were deliberating.

"You want to know what the problem is? I miss Andrea. I missed her the whole time we were gone. I've never felt this way about anyone—including you. I feel something for her that I've never felt for you, and I never will."

That was it. A few years ago this would have crushed me. Now it enraged me.

"Get up. Get out of bed now and go to Andrea. We are not married anymore. I'm not your wife anymore. This marriage is over."

Michael didn't move.

"Get out, Michael!" I screamed.

He stormed off to the living room, slamming the door behind him. I jumped out of bed and locked it so he couldn't return. I was too angry to sleep. I stomped around our small bedroom. I looked at the drawer where I had found Meg's letters years earlier. That was the beginning of the end, I thought. Then I started crying. These were tears of grief. I was mourning a marriage that was irreversibly, unmistakably dead. At around 3 AM I finally faded into a short, fitful sleep.

When I woke the alarm clock read 5:15 and the dawn was gradually bathing the bedroom in a soft light. I was sad, but also relieved. Now it was out in the open and any lingering doubts or misguided hopes about salvaging the relationship were extinguished. I had come to the marriage with a fantasy about where it would lead and what it would be like. I made Michael into who I wanted him to be, not who he was. There had been wonderful times, to be sure. We'd raised two kind, bright, beautiful kids together, and on some level I would always love Michael. But, after three decades together, I had to face the fact that the marriage was never what I had told myself it was, and Michael was never the husband I had created in my mind. That was an illusion—one that I had crafted, and I was now ready to let it go.

I walked out into the living room and found Michael sitting up on the sofa. He turned his head when he heard my footsteps. Dark circles shadowed his eyes and his hair looked like it had been through a cyclone.

I almost felt sorry for him, but I wasn't backing down.

"Cheryl, I didn't mean it. I was just trying to hurt you."

"Anybody who would do that to me . . . talk to me like that after all the years we've been together. I can't be with you anymore, Michael."

I looked out our back window at the cottage that sat on our property. It had come with the house when we bought it in 1978. The only question now was how soon Michael would move into it. Within the week Michael had packed up his books, records, clothes, and other belongings and decamped to the backyard.

℘

By April 1993, Michael and I had lived as neighbors for almost a year, and had settled into a kind of friendship. Bob stayed with me several nights a week, and Andrea lived intermittently with Michael. When Jessica and Eric came, we got together in the house that I had now assumed full ownership of and had dinner, watched movies, or just hung out together. As I acquired some distance from Michael, I also gained clarity. Michael had brought his own issues to the marriage. I no longer believed that he couldn't love me because I wasn't good enough. Instead I saw how he'd always battled his own insecurities and demons. I wasn't sure he could love any woman. This helped me to have some compassion for him and to dial back my anger enough for a friendship to grow.

Financial circumstances didn't allow Michael to move from the backyard bungalow. In fact, I chuckled when the judge at our separation hearing asked me if I was sure about not going after him for spousal support. I just hope he doesn't go after me, I thought. He didn't, and when it came time to divvy up the few assets I had cobbled together as the major wage earner of the family, he demanded little. If we were going to be neighbors, we would try to be good ones for our own well-being and for the sake of our children.

I think I would have felt pretty good if it wasn't for the almost constant pain I now had in my stomach. When it started I attributed it to stress. Some days it was so intense that I couldn't eat. I had dropped a few stubborn pounds, and even though I felt terrible, I was getting close to the body I had wanted for years. If I could only maintain the diet the pain imposed on me after it was gone, I thought, I could stay slim into my fifth decade. The problem was that the pain didn't go away. It kept me up at night and stopped me from working. After one particularly bad day in July 1993, when I was unable to get out of bed and could barely take a drink of water, I called my doctor and said I needed to come in immediately.

"Sounds like diverticulitis," said Dr. Sanders, who, at the time, was seven months pregnant. She prescribed antibiotics and said she would get me an appointment with a gastroenterologist if I didn't improve.

A week later I was still in agony and called Dr. Sanders. She had left for maternity leave, but her nurse gave me the name and phone number for Dr. Jedson, a local gastroenterologist, who, mercifully, had an opening that afternoon.

Dr. Jedson had a soft-spoken, calm manner that put me at ease instantly. The medication I had been taking made so little difference to my condition that I had begun to doubt the diverticulitis diagnosis. This guy is going to figure out what's really wrong with me, I thought with relief. After he examined me, he announced that I would need to get a CAT scan—the following morning. I wanted to know what was wrong with me, but this seemed awfully fast. Doesn't it take at least a day to navigate the medical bureaucracy? Should I be worried? I asked Dr. Jedson where I should go to make the appointment, and he said he had already made it for me. Now I really was worried. It seemed like I was getting special treatment and this was not a context in which I wanted to be special.

I phoned Bob, who immediately called his work to tell them he wouldn't be in the next day. I also told Michael, who immediately volunteered to join us. He was genuinely concerned. After all we had been through, Michael and I still had a bond, and I had to admit I wanted him there. I needed all the support I could get, and if he wasn't a reliable husband, Michael was turning into a supportive friend.

The following morning the three of us reported to a lab in downtown Berkeley. I left Michael and Bob chatting amiably in the waiting room and followed a nurse down a corridor that led to the large room that housed the donut-shaped CAT scan machine.

I lay down on what looked like a chute protruding out of the machine. The tech told me to hold my breath when I saw the green light on the rim of the scanner. I heard what sounded like a vacuum cleaner being used in a distant room as I glided backward into the tunnel of the machine. The green light went on and I caught my breath. Then several mysterious clicks, and the green light flipped off. A minute later it was on again and the clicks returned. We did this five or six times.

I returned to the waiting room and sat between Michael and Bob. If I hadn't been so anxious about what the test might reveal, I probably would have been coming up with a way to explain to the doctor who the two men with me were. I chuckled at the idea of introducing Bob as my future husband, since Reno didn't count legally, and Michael as my future ex-husband. In as soon as a few minutes I would learn what was behind the excruciating pain that had dogged me for the last two months. I was afraid of what the test might reveal, but looked forward to finally undergoing the treatment that would alleviate the agony and let me get on with my life.

It looks like I have a rain cloud in my stomach, I thought as the three of us looked up at the scan of my abdomen that was pressed against a light box on the wall of an exam room. "See all this grey?" the doctor said. "That's your lymph system. You have lymphoma.

These are all tumors." I heard him, but I didn't really assimilate what he said. Lymphoma was cancer, and I couldn't have cancer. I looked at Bob and then at Michael. They both looked as serious as I had ever seen them. The doctor took out a prescription pad and scribbled the name and number of an oncologist on it. He held it out toward me, but I just stood there. Finally, Bob took it from him. We walked silently to the car. Bob opened the door for me and I got into the passenger side. Bob didn't normally do this. It struck me how terribly grave my situation really was.

∾

Dr. Resner, the oncologist, was a slender man with a gentle demeanor. His black hair was dusted with grey at the temples and he had a lilting voice. He explained that I had tumors from just below my heart to my groin. They were crowded around my stomach and many of my organs. This was why I couldn't eat and why I was in so much pain. He needed to do a number of blood tests and other exams before he could tell me how we should proceed. First, I would have surgical biopsy to remove some swollen lymph nodes. This would tell them which of the many varieties of lymphoma I had. A bone marrow test would follow, and when he had all of the results, we would reconvene.

On a late July morning, Bob, Michael, Jessica, Eric, and I climbed into Michael's car and drove across town to the hospital. I had to be there at 6 AM to check in for surgery and we were a bleary-eyed bunch. The surgery would be done under general anesthesia, and if all went well it wouldn't take longer than two hours. The surgeon would make an incision above my right collar bone and extract the lymph nodes.

When we arrived, Jessica and Eric headed to the cafeteria for coffee while I completed a stack of forms. Soon I had an ID bracelet clamped around my wrist and had changed into a blue hospital gown. A friendly nurse prepped me and the surgeon arrived and asked if I had any questions. One by one my beautiful family kissed me and assured me they would be there when I awoke. The last thing I remember is counting aloud to ten after the anesthesiologist covered my nose and mouth with a mask.

The barely perceptible weight of the breathing tube resting below my nose was the first thing I felt when I resurfaced. An IV line sprung out of my arm, and I could hear faint chattering coming from the nurses' station outside my door. Next to the lower right corner of my bed Jessica was slumped forward in a chair, her arms on the bed and her head resting on her arms. Droll, whip-smart, and artistic, Jessica was a born rebel and I couldn't be prouder to be her mother.

"Jess, what's wrong, honey?"

"What's wrong? What's wrong? You're in the hospital. You have cancer. You're knocking your forehead on the threshold of Monsieur Reaper," she said in the most exaggerated French accent I had ever heard.

A spasm of pain rippled across the surgical cut and I felt the stitches pull.

"Don't make me laugh," I said, and pursed my lips to staunch any more giggling.

With the support of my loving, quirky family and friends I hoped to send Monsieur Reaper packing.

What, exactly, the grim reaper threatened me with became clearer after the surgery and other tests. I had follicular mixed-cell low-grade lymphoma. It was in stage three, not the best time for detection, but not as dire as stages four or five. The cancer had not gone into my bone marrow, and, if I followed the treatment protocol, I had a 95 percent chance of shrinking the tumors. Survival rates for this kind of cancer were high.

I needed to hear this. I was still in tremendous discomfort, even though I now had a steady supply of painkillers, and I was weak and exhausted. I was still unable to eat and had lost thirty pounds. At times I thought I would rather die than continue on in this kind of misery. My resolve was running thin. There were days when I could barely hold my chin up. For the first time I realized the weight of my head. It felt like I had a bowling ball balanced atop my neck. Still, my prognosis was positive.

Dr. Resner explained that I would be treated with something called CHOP, a chemotherapy regimen that includes cylcophosphamide, hydroxydaunorubicin, oncovin, and prednisone. Three weeks earlier I had never heard of these drugs. Their impenetrable names scared me. I wanted to go back to the time when I didn't know the word *chop* could be an acronym. Still, my prognosis was positive.

⁀

When the chemo started I would lose my hair that hung to the middle of my back. I decided that at the first sign of hair loss I would shave my head. It was a way of reclaiming some degree of power over a body that had spun out of control. I also vowed to devote all of my energy to my recovery. Squandering any of it on anger or bitterness was a luxury I could no longer afford. I had to concentrate on getting well as quickly as possible. I already had to take time off and turn away potential clients because I was too sick to work. I knew I would not be able to work as I went through treatment and that I would have to dip into my scant savings to make ends meet.

I vowed that I would care for myself as best as I could. Michael and I had studied hypnosis together a few years earlier and he agreed to hypnotize me every day. I made an appointment with a nutritionist and doubled up on my psychotherapy visits. A former client heard I was sick and he arranged for a massage therapist to visit me after every chemo treatment. Bob cashed in the five months of vacation time he had accrued as a postal worker for the last ten years, and barely left my side. Both Jessica and Eric were at the ready to help whenever I needed it. My support network was sturdy and reliable, not just because of who was in it, but because of who wasn't.

I decided that I wouldn't call my parents as I went through treatment. Against my wishes, Michael had told them about my diagnosis shortly after I had received it. I didn't want them to know that I was miserable. Almost three decades after I had left for California and began a life with Michael, they still expected disaster to strike. I didn't want to prove them right. Michael told me that they took it in their typical stoic manner and asked him to call if I took a turn for the worse. No great outpourings of sympathy flowed from them. Hasty travel plans to visit me in California were not made. So be it. My plan was to avoid anyone who didn't support or comfort or relax me, and if that meant temporarily cutting off my parents, then that's what I would do.

With chemotherapy looming, I thought carefully about what I needed to forgive others and myself for if I was going to muster every bit of my energy for healing. As I well knew, anger and resentment were parasites that could quickly drain away precious internal resources. I worked on forgiving Michael, and forgiving myself for putting up with him. If my mind alighted on a memory that sparked anger, I reminded myself that my energy was now to be used in the service of getting well. On some days I had to tell myself this only once; on others I had to say it repeatedly. Before my diagnosis, the thought of extending an olive branch to Meg would have seemed about as plausible as walking on water. Now, it felt almost necessary, so a few days before I was due to begin chemo I called her.

"Cheryl, is that you?" Meg asked when I said hello.

"It's me, Meg."

There was a long pause.

"Well, I suppose Michael has told you that I'm . . . I'm sick. Well, I mean I have lymphoma and I'm going start chemo soon."

"He did, Cheryl. I'm sorry," Meg said in a timorous voice. Maybe she thought I was calling to release my anger, which I was, but not in the way she might have suspected.

"Meg, it's okay," I said.

"Thanks. It's hard to know what to say."

"I'm calling today because I want you to know that I'm not angry with you. If I die—and I don't plan to—I don't want you feeling like I died hating you. I understand what happened. You're a human being. We all are, and we fell in love with the same person."

"Cheryl, I'm sorry for . . . for a lot, but I can't say I'm sorry for having my kids."

"I don't want you to apologize for that. I love your kids and I'm glad they're in my life."

Forgiveness doesn't happen in the course of one phone call, but it was a beginning. And I believed Meg. She hadn't intended to hurt me, and even if she had, I was doing my best to jettison anger—no exceptions.

"No exceptions" included my parents too. For a long time I dreamed of a reconciliation with them that would consist of more than a series of tacit agreements not to talk about what we knew would trigger a fight. I wanted them to accept and love me for who I was. I wanted them to rethink much of what they believed, and I wanted them to understand how much their attitudes about sexuality had hurt me. I yearned for them to recognize me as a loving mother, a competent professional, and even a good daughter. I also realized that I was in no position to set contingencies and conditions on forgiveness. I had to let my anger toward them dissipate no matter what they had or hadn't done, and that's what I committed to finally do. It wasn't the closure I wanted, but it was the one I had to accept.

Bob and Michael arranged to accompany me to my first chemotherapy infusion appointment. For his part, Michael had continued to make a diligent effort at friendship and I welcomed it. "It's complicated" is used flippantly these days, but our relationship was . . . well . . . complicated. Michael and I had essentially grown up together: We had raised children together and experimented together. Our shared history, however tumultuous, would keep us in each other's lives. Michael would stand beside me as I faced the worst health crisis of my life. If the situation were reversed, I would have been there for him, with all of my anger and love, resentment and tenderness. He attended the first three chemo sessions.

"Does she ever . . . " I heard Michael whisper to Bob just as I had settled in to my first chemotherapy infusion. He shot me a mischievous look. I appreciated the attempt at a joke, but I was in no mood to laugh.

"Oh God, could you please not do that," I said.

Bob went back to his photography magazine and Michael stared out the window. I didn't need them comparing notes while drip-by-drip I took in the toxins that would save my life. Including this one, I was scheduled for six treatments, one every three weeks. It was August, and if all went as planned I would be done by Christmas, and I'd begin 1994 cancer-free.

I reclined back, closed my eyes, and thought about the Grand Canyon and Europe, two places I wanted to see more desperately than ever. When I regained my health I was going to make those trips a priority. It may sound clichéd, but having cancer forced me to realize that I didn't have all the time in the world to do what I wanted to do. Procrastination was now the enemy.

As treatment wound on, I was thankful for many things. My family and friends were at the top of my list. Zofran, an antinausea drug that was relatively new at the time, was second. After my first infusion, my stomach felt like it was on spin cycle. Morning sickness was nothing compared to this. I vomited until I had nothing left in me and I was so weak that I had to be virtually carried the twenty feet from my bathroom to my bedroom. After that, I took Zofran intravenously before every treatment and in pill form if I needed it afterward.

Most of the time I was so exhausted that I had to remind myself that I was on my way to getting well. It sure didn't feel like it. On my own I wouldn't have left the house much, but my family took turns getting me out. More than once I heard one of my kids say, "Let's take Mom for a walk." If I had had the strength I would have laughed. What was I, a dog?

Bob also got me out. Once we took a trip to the University of California's Botanical Gardens, where we had our first date. We walked along a path, Bob supporting me at each step. I soon had to rest and sat on the nearest bench. I put my head on Bob's shoulder. I closed my eyes for a few minutes and almost fell asleep. Then I heard a child giggling. I looked up and coming toward us was a toddler tootling along, his beaming parents rushing to keep up with him. He had a head full of brown curls and bright blue eyes. He tried to climb up a little dirt mound, and when he lost his footing he slid down laughing. His mother brushed the dirt off his knees and kissed his chubby cheeks.

He's just starting his life, I thought. That was me at one time. His parents are just starting their lives with him. That was once me, too. I may be at the end of my life. I felt enormous sadness for myself, and boundless joy for the strangers who walked toward me. How quickly life can end. It can all be over in a flash. I closed my eyes tight so Bob wouldn't see me cry. Look at how much you've had, I said to myself. People younger than you die all the time all over the world. Children die. Babies die. They live for less time than a butterfly. You've had a good life, a rich life with so much experience. It's going to be okay if you die. When I opened my eyes the family was gone, slipped away in the span of a few thoughts.

I don't like the word *remission*, probably because of its sister word, *recurrence*. I prefer to think of myself as cured, and that's what I told Dr. Resner on the last of our appointments. The chemo had done its job, and I could return to life and work. The anger and resentment I had accumulated over the years was also gone. I had a man who loved me, a newly healthy body, and a deeper appreciation of what mattered in life. At fifty, I had learned volumes—enough to make the next half-century even better than the first.

19.

sex and the senior girl: esther

···

As I entered the new millennium, most of my crowd was either firmly ensconced in the senior citizen bracket or on the cusp of it. The generation who venerated youth was doing the impossible—getting old—and this meant coming to terms with our aging bodies and changes to our sexuality.

After the Dalkon Shield disaster in my twenties, a thick layer of scar tissue built up in my fallopian tubes and my ovaries were covered in cysts. Between forty and forty-six, I had three operations to remove them. I resisted the surgeries for as long as I could and refused my doctor's advice to have a complete hysterectomy because I knew that it would affect my libido. When one of my doctors asked why I needed my uterus, since I wasn't going to have children, it betrayed a shocking ignorance about female sexuality. I explained that not having my uterus would limit my ability to have orgasms. My uterus was still perfectly healthy and removing it would shorten my vagina and needlessly impact my sex life. He argued that it would protect me from uterine cancer, but I wasn't going to have it removed for preventative reasons. I wondered how he would feel about preemptive testicle removal. Would he volunteer for that to protect himself from testicular cancer?

Regardless, I had three surgeries to remove my fallopian tubes and ovaries, and I did worry about how this would affect my libido. And I would find out, because after the surgeries, my hormonal balance shifted and my libido became a shadow of what it was. I decided to go on hormone replacement therapy, and to rely on my decades of solid sex education. I knew that communication, imagination, and a willingness to experiment go a long way toward turning up the erotic temperature. If my body's thermostat had been reset, my thought process would have to contribute more.

Sexual energy took longer to ignite, and while I still had orgasms, they no longer felt like a tidal wave sweeping through my body. I had to go to the ultimate source: my brain. I dipped into my treasure trove of sexy memories and relied more on fantasy to kick-start arousal. I reminded myself that sexuality changes over the course of a lifetime, and I was no exception. It was time for me to take the advice that I had given to friends and clients countless times: Keep playing; keep experimenting.

~

When I was in my early sixties I had an experience that inspired me to charge into my older years with as much commitment to having satisfying sex as ever. Esther was an old friend who had recently turned eighty-four. Married for over half a century, her husband, Henry, now struggled with dementia, arthritis, and a number of other conditions that spelled an end to his sex life. Esther loved and cared for Henry, and she was determined to revive her sex life.

She didn't come to me as a client, but as a friend who wanted the benefit of my expertise.

One Saturday she came over for brunch. We sat in my backyard enjoying the first flowers of spring, sipping mimosas, and eating eggs and croissants. Esther explained that she wasn't ready to walk away from the exhilarating sex she had enjoyed for much of her married life. She referred to her orgasms with Henry as "earthquakes, but good ones." She wanted to return to them, or at least feel pleasure and arousal, but she needed a little help learning how to achieve this on her own.

"Here's where you come in, Cheryl," she said. When she flashed her lovely grin, a group of wrinkles gathered around her mouth.

"How can I help?"

"I want to learn more about sex toys. I tried a vibrator years ago, but I didn't like it. Can we take a trip to that store?"

"Good Vibrations?"

"Yes, that's the one."

I wish every town had a store like Good Vibrations. It's a boutique that offers sex toys, lubes, condoms, books, movies, games, and more. They were founded on sex-positive principles and have helpful, knowledgeable staff who make everyone feel welcome. I remembered how exciting it was when they opened in 1977, and we suddenly had a classy community sex store that we could patronize without hesitation or shame.

Esther and I had drained our mimosas and finished our leisurely meal and decided we'd visit Good Vibrations the following day.

                             ℘

When I arrived at Esther's house the next morning, she had pulled her gunmetal grey hair back into a knot, and wore rose-colored lipstick.

"The big day," she said.

We headed over to the Berkeley store, and as we drove I gave her a preview of what she would find there.

"They have lots of vibrators and dildos, and just about everything you need to go with them. How is your lubrication these days? Do you think you might need something to help with it?"

"That's another thing. I've gotten very dry."

"Okay. That happens to many women after menopause, and most women at your age have a lot of dryness. We'll take a look. My advice is to try a few different samples and see what works best."

I parked around the corner, helped Esther out of the car, and we made our way to the store.

"Whoa," Esther said, her hazel eyes wide, as we walked through the front door.

She scanned the large room and only moved out from the entryway when she realized a few people had circled around her to get in.

I gave Esther a quick tour. Dildos, vibrators, and other toys were on one side of the room; lubes, massage oils, and additional items were on the other. Just then an employee recognized me and said hello. I introduced her to Esther and told her it was her first trip to the store.

"Welcome, Esther. Let me know if I can help with anything," she said.

"Thank you, dear," Esther replied, still a little bedazzled.

I showed Esther my favorite lube and gave her my take on others. I doubt she heard much of what I said because her eyes were focused on the other side of the room where a huge variety of dildos and vibrators were affixed to the far wall.

"See anything interesting?" I asked.

"I think so. I'm going to take a look over there," Esther said and, cane in hand, she made her way to the sex toys.

I busied myself with checking out the lubricants, condoms, and other supplies. I needed to stock up for both work and home. Just as I had put a few boxes of condoms in my hand basket, I looked up and saw Esther smiling at me from across the room. She was holding an almost foot-long, blue, silicone dildo.

I walked over to her.

"That one looks good?"

"I'd like to give a try. Tell me, Cheryl, do you have a preference?"

For years I had used a vibrator that was probably three-quarters the size of the one Esther grasped in her hand. As I had aged, however, I discovered I loved the Pocket Rocket vibrator, which was considerably smaller, about four inches long, and had one only speed, but it was a little powerhouse.

"Let me show you what I like these days," I said.

We went to the toy shelf and I pointed out the Pocket Rocket.

"It's good for traveling, too," I said.

"But it's so small."

"Well, you don't need to go very deep to be stimulated."

"Hmm . . . I always liked big men, and Harry got huge when he was ready," Esther said.

She looked at the behemoth in her hand and then at the Pocket Rocket on the shelf.

"I think I'll try both."

"Good idea. Experiment with them and see what you like best."

She picked out a few different kinds of lube and we headed to the cash register.

Esther and I had a quick bite to eat and then I drove her home.

She called the next weekend. I didn't take much prompting to get her report.

"How are you doing?" I asked.

"Oh, Cheryl, that Pocket Rocket. Maybe I've overestimated size or maybe I've changed, but, whoa, it's my new best friend."

Her comment reminded me of an incident in my early twenties. I was visiting with a friend who lived with her mother and grandmother. Her great aunt happened to also be visiting the day I was there, and the two elderly sisters sat in the kitchen within earshot of my friend and me in the living room.

"I'm so glad that's over," I heard one of them say.

"Me too. It's such a relief that he doesn't want it anymore," the other one answered.

I realized they were talking about sex. My friend and I looked at each other. "I hope we never feel like that," I said.

Now, listening to Esther sing the praises of her new Pocket Rocket, I was sure I wouldn't. I was also certain that my generation, the one that had turned the world upside down in the sixties and seventies, wasn't going to abandon sex because of age. Our bodies change as we grow older, but that just means we have to find new ways of being sexual. Along with my grey-haired friends and colleagues, I was writing a new chapter of my sex life, not an epilogue.

20.

still cooking

....

"**C**heryl, you need to come over here right away." Sarah sounded like she could barely breathe enough to push the words out. My heart pumped so hard that I could feel it reverberate in my ears and arms. This had to be bad. "Is Eric dead?" I asked. It was the worst news I could imagine my daughter-in-law delivering. "No, no, but you need to come over here now."

It was 2001 and my son, his wife, and my young grandchild lived in the cottage in my backyard. Michael had vacated a few years earlier to set up house with Jan, his latest girlfriend.

I jammed my feet into a pair of flip-flops and flew down the back steps and down the path that separated our houses, my legs powered by the adrenaline that raced through me. As I bounded up the front stairs, I lost one of my shoes.

"What, what is it?" I asked Sarah.

"Cheryl, I have bad news. Michael is dead."

"Michael who?" I asked, not able to comprehend that it could be my Michael.

"Michael Cohen," she answered.

I felt like I had been walloped with a two-by-four.

"What? Oh, oh my God," I gasped.

Michael's birthday was three days away. On February 3 he would have been sixty-one.

"Eric is on his way home. I called him at work," she said.

"What happened?"

"He had a massive heart attack at school. Jan called. She's at the hospital."

Michael had been working as a special education teacher. It was the first time he had held a steady job in years. He was popular with the students and had achieved notable success with even some of the most challenging ones. The principal of the school was stunned at the change he had seen in some of the kids.

How could he be dead? The notion of Michael no longer walking the planet seemed impossible. All of his knowledge and ideas and feelings and passions and craziness were gone. I would never see him again. Michael, the man who had changed my life, was no more. The man with whom I had fallen in and out of love, the one who had infuriated me, who had given me two beautiful children, who had made me laugh, who had betrayed me, was dead. I would never talk to him again. How could it be?

I sat down on the sofa and put my head in my hands. I tried to calm myself as I looked down at my one naked foot.

"I can't believe it. I can't believe it," I said to Sarah and myself.

I thought about calling Jessica at work, but I called her best friend Ellen instead.

Ellen and Jessica were like sisters, and I wanted her there with me when I broke the sad news. I was in no shape to drive, so Ellen picked me up and we left for the jewelry store where Jessica worked.

Jessica's face lit up when she saw the two of us enter the store and then quickly dropped when she registered my expression.

"What's wrong?" she asked

"Jessica, honey. Something really sad has happened. Your father died."

"Oh, Mom. Are you okay?" was the first thing my sweet daughter said to me after I told her.

She came out from behind the counter to hug me. I felt her burning face and her tears through my shirt.

"If I'd only known it would be the last time I'd see him . . . " she said.

We walked out to the parking lot with our arms around each other and Ellen drove us home.

I called Bob, who was now officially my husband. In 1995, we exchanged wedding vows, again, in front of about fifty family and friends. He got in his car the minute we hung up and soon all of us were standing in my son's living room.

Jan had identified the body, but we decided we would all go to the hospital morgue. It was as if we all required proof that Michael was dead.

When we arrived, Bob stayed in the hospital lobby with my eleven-month-old granddaughter while the rest of us got in the elevator and descended to the morgue.

The fluorescent light gleamed off of the rows of stainless steel drawers. It was all so cold and impersonal, so uniform. A revolving door of grief swept the ones left behind in and out. It was our turn now. It would be someone else's tomorrow.

The coroner slid one of the drawers open and there lay Michael. I felt like I was going to faint. The blood had pooled toward the back of his body, and I glimpsed a sliver of purple under his ear. His skin was waxen and his eyes were shut, permanently.

"Oh, Daddy," Jessica said.

I started crying for myself, for Jessica, for all of us. We each took turns saying goodbye. When it was mine, I knelt down on the floor and kissed Michael's cold lips. I touched his face and chest. How the fuck did this happen? I thought. I felt guilty, like I shouldn't be as upset as I was. Michael was no longer my husband and I had a wonderful partner in Bob. Was I being disloyal to him? I'm so sorry, Michael, I whispered.

Then we walked out, each of us reaching for the hand that was closest.

I often wonder how Michael and I would have interacted with the benefit of age and hindsight. Since our divorce, Michael had talked more openly about his emotions and fears than he ever had during our marriage. He once said to me that he marveled at how every time life knocked me down I got back up again. "I wouldn't be able to do that. I would just curl up in a ball to try to protect myself," he said. He also admitted that he had never been able to give me the kind of intimacy I wanted. "You loved me so fiercely that it scared me. I was afraid of losing your love, of letting you down." He wanted to work on himself, to face his fears, and to lower the barriers that kept him from fully loving any woman.

How sad for Michael, I thought. He had so many gifts and so many adoring women in his life, but he missed out on so much by not being able to love. I saw then that, in a way, he had always been alone.

The year after Michael died I lost another person whose impact on me was profound. In 2002, at seventy-seven, my mother died of bone cancer.

After I recovered from lymphoma, I came to a crossroads with Mom. My commitment to staying as positive and stress-free as possible was tested every time we talked. Our conversations typically ended with me sobbing and angry. I was convinced that if I was going to stay healthy, I had to steer clear of the toxic emotions that contact with my mother invariably generated. So, I decided that she and I would change how we interacted or we would no longer speak.

One Saturday in 1995 I made a phone call that changed our relationship. "Mom, I can't keep doing this," I said. I had practiced what

I would say to her for days, and I was confident. "We need to change," I continued. There was total silence on the other end. For a minute I thought she had hung up, but then I heard her sigh. Keep going, I told myself. "We can't continue pushing each other's buttons. It upsets you and me, and it's not healthy for either one of us. I want us to let go of the past. You'll always be my mother, but now I want to see if we can be friends. When we talk to each other, I want us to stay in the present. Who knows how much longer either one of us has in this life. Let's not spend it being angry at each other. We can't change the past, but we can make a different future for ourselves. I forgive you and I want you to forgive me."

"What have you got to forgive me for?"

I felt a twinge of anger, and reminded myself that I had just suggested that we leave the past behind us.

"Mom, I'm not going to go there. Let's stay in the present. No more rehashing the past. If you can't do this, I can't speak to you anymore."

My mother was quiet.

"I want you to really think about this," I said.

After we hung up I didn't know if I had talked to my mother for the last time. I had worked hard to forgive her and to let go of the rage and resentment that had hung on since childhood. I wasn't willing to have it rekindled with every phone call.

It was about a week until I heard from my mother again. For the first time in several years, she sent me a letter instead of calling.

When Mom left for Mass on the Sunday morning after our talk, she was rankled. She had done her best as a mother and had worked hard. Why was I so mad at her? Shouldn't she be the one with a grudge? Was my childhood so terrible? After all, I had never wanted for anything. She was still fuming when the priest began his sermon, which was on forgiveness. He talked about how Jesus Christ had set the example of forgiveness, and about how healing begins with it. It was our duty, and even our salvation, to forgive.

Somewhere in the course of the homily, the idea of calling a truce with me started to seem at first possible, then desirable. By the time she left the church she had started to think more deeply about what I had said. Maybe, after all these years, it was time to move on. She waited a few days before starting the letter to me. "I want to try what you suggested," she wrote.

My mother and I vowed to put aside the rancor and resentment and forge a new relationship. When we talked we would stay in the present and not relive past hurts, slights, and traumas. We would side-step topics that we knew would ignite arguments. I had gripes with her as a mother, and she was never shy when it came to her complaints about me as a daughter, but we were both adults now. It was time to see if we could transcend the bitterness and become friends.

To my great surprise and delight, my mother and I were able to begin again. We found that we actually enjoyed each other's company and our bond grew and deepened over the last seven years of her life. She even opened up to me about her sex life. Turns out my father was a wonderful lover, who always made sure she was "satisfied." Sure, it was more information than I wanted, but it was also a yardstick that measured just how much our relationship had changed.

Incredibly, there was only one time when mom brought up the past by mentioning her anger at Michael. When I asked her to let it go and stay in the present, she did without an argument. I was grateful to my mother for her efforts and willingness to change. Anger had become a habit for both of us, and it was difficult to break away from the old patterns and the familiar dynamic, but she did it. When I lost her in 2002, I lost a friend.

‌‌‌
_⁓_

By 2006, Bob and I had shared our lives for twenty-seven years. There had been many good times and a few bad, and we delighted in the former and weathered the latter as a team. In the winter of that year, life would throw us yet another curve ball. It had been almost thirteen years since my brush with cancer and, to my shock, it was now back. This time it was in my breast.

I had a small lump on my right areola that my radiologist initially speculated was a blocked milk duct. A mammogram picked up a number of tiny, suspicious-looking spots, but no one used the c-word yet. I was told to have another mammogram in six months. "We'll keep an eye on it," the radiologist said. I trusted her judgment and left the hospital relieved. Six months later when I dutifully returned for the follow-up screening, I was advised that nothing had changed and that the best course would be to remain vigilant and continue with semi-annual mammograms. Once again, I went about my life confident that I was in no imminent danger. Coincidentally, a few days after my second test, my old pal Barbara, a fellow surrogate, called to tell me that our mutual friend, another Barbara, had undergone a lumpectomy after being diagnosed with breast cancer. As soon as we hung up I called the other Barbara to see how she was recovering. We chatted for a bit and I asked what her symptoms were. "Well, at first they told me I had a blocked milk duct," she said.

The next call I made was to Evelyn, another surrogate, who had had a mastectomy several years earlier. I explained my situation, and she gave me what in retrospect was the best advice I could have received. "Tell them you want a stereotactic biopsy." Within a week I had an appointment for one, and for a biopsy of the lump on my areola.

When Dr. Whitney walked into the exam room she had a serious look on her narrow face.

"I have breast cancer, don't I?" I said.

"Yes, you do."

I had infiltrating ductal carcinoma. She sat down and spread out the results from the stereotactic biopsy across her lap.

I felt like I was hovering above my body as I watched the scene play out.

"I'm going to take the biopsy of the lump. I'll have the lab analyze it and we'll get the results in about twenty minutes. Lie down and relax and I'll be back soon."

"I'm fine," I said in disbelief.

"Cheryl, you're in shock. Lie down and when I have the results we'll take all the time we need to go over them and decide what to do," Dr. Whitney said.

I lay down, but as soon as the door closed I jumped up and pulled my phone out of my purse.

I dialed my friend Joanne's number. "I have cancer. I have cancer—again," I told her, trembling.

"Come over here as soon as you can," she said.

Then I phoned the nutritionist I had worked with when I had lymphoma.

"Have them send me all of your lab work. I'll put together a plan for you. We'll work together like we did before," she told me, concerned but firm.

I was instinctively, immediately reaching out to my support system. Once again, I resolved to do everything I could to survive. I put away my phone and eased back on the exam table, crinkling the paper that lay over it. I took slow, deep breaths until Dr. Whitney returned.

She did a needle biopsy on the lump and soon we were discussing how we would treat the now undeniable cancer in my breast. The cancer in the lump was the same as that in my breast, which is not always the case. I learned that there are over forty different kinds of breast cancer and women can have more than one type simultaneously. Infiltrating ductal carcinoma is one of the most treatable, especially when caught in stage one, as was the case for me.

"I would recommend a mastectomy, given the number of small tumors," Dr. Whitney said.

The mysterious spots that the mammograms had picked up were actually tiny, one-millimeter tumors clustered together in one quadrant of my breast. They were so small that at first Dr. Whitney could barely make them out.

"Fine. Should I let you take the other breast too?"

I wanted the cancer gone and I wanted any chance of cancer in my other breast to go along with it. I didn't like the prospect of losing both breasts, but I liked the possibility of having to undergo treatment again even less, and in that moment my suggestion seemed logical.

Dr. Whitney assured me that I had a relatively low chance of developing cancer in my left breast and that only the right needed to be removed. When they performed the mastectomy, they would take out a few of my lymph nodes to be sure the cancer had not spread to them.

I asked her if this cancer was related to the lymphoma I had survived years earlier and she answered with an emphatic no.

One of the first things I did when I got home was find a breast cancer support group. I had joined a group after my lymphoma diagnosis and had found it to be a powerful adjunct to my treatment.

$\wp$

I had my mastectomy in February 2006. Luckily, the cancer had not spread to my lymph nodes and I wouldn't need chemotherapy or radiation. I was sent home with two drainage bulbs dangling from my right side, below my armpit. I had to measure the amount of fluid in them every day so they could see that it was diminishing. I also had a fluid-filled flexible plastic expander in my chest to prepare my skin for reconstructive surgery, which would take place in April. Once a week I visited the reconstructive surgeon to have fluid added to the expander so that my skin wouldn't contract. Most of the time I was uncomfortable, but I was rarely in pain. Apart from the first day or two after the surgery, I didn't even take the Percocet that had been prescribed for me.

The mastectomy impacted my body image significantly. I'd grown to accept and love my breasts, even though they weren't the perky mounds I had always wanted. I loved having my nipples sucked and played with during sex. The reconstruction would bring my shape back into balance, but I knew that the sensitivity in my right side would be much less than what I was accustomed to feeling.

I had to remind myself that I was more than my breasts. When I finally said it out loud to a friend it seemed so obvious that I hardly had to repeat it to myself or anyone else. In a way I had to relearn what I had discovered in my modeling days: An imperfect body could still be a sexy body. True, I would have to accept a loss of sensation, but I still had plenty of ways to receive pleasure.

Fortunately, Bob, once again, proved to be a supportive and devoted partner. When he learned that the cancer hadn't spread into my lymph nodes his relief was on par with mine. He nursed me throughout my recovery, and our intimate life stayed strong. He often told me that all he wanted was for me to regain my health and that the worst thing he could imagine was that I would feel that I was somehow less appealing to him.

As I looked forward to the reconstruction, I began to think more about how the change in my body would affect my work. My greatest concern was that it would shift the focus of my interaction with a client to me, when it should be on him. I believed that clients needed to know about the mastectomy because my right breast would look and feel different from my left, and I didn't want them to be distracted by that. One day I brought up my fear in my support group. Dr. Renaldi, one of two psychotherapists who led the group, asked me how I thought I should address the issue with clients. Having the opportunity to talk out a plan was exactly what I needed at this time. I decided that I wouldn't mention it in the earliest part of the work when I was interviewing the client about his history, issues, and goals. I would reveal it only when we moved to the bedroom, and I would discuss it matter-of-factly. No great announcements, just another item on the checklist of need-to-know information. If I didn't want a client to overly focus on my mastectomy, I had to be sure I kept it in perspective too.

I had another question that wouldn't be answered so easily. I struggled with how I would talk about my breasts in the mirror exercise. Cancer would become part of the story of my body. Lymphoma may have been a more frightening diagnosis and a more grueling recovery, but my body had remained externally intact after it. Now, when I stood before a full-length mirror with a client following along, I would have to address the differences in my breasts. The new vocabulary I would need for this was nowhere in sight, but I had a feeling it would come in time, as I healed.

∽

The reconstructive surgery didn't even keep me in the hospital overnight. To help me look more even, the surgeon lifted my left breast and moved the nipple slightly upward. A silicone implant went into my right side.

It didn't take long to realize that the surgery was a success. Under a bra and blouse my breasts looked even and unremarkable. When I undressed the difference between the two was evident, but not startling. What was more complicated was coming to terms with the loss of sensation. My new right breast had some faint sensitivity, but that was it. Once it healed I had to decide if I wanted, for aesthetic reasons, to have a nipple constructed from surrounding tissue. The appearance of my new breast sans nipple was fine with me, so I opted to pass on it.

One of the many lessons I have learned from working with disabled people is the importance of focusing on what you can feel and experience, as opposed to dwelling on limitations. Doing away with preconceived notions about how and where you should feel pleasure and training your attention on where you do feel it can sometimes make you forget that you have nonreactive areas. I'd seen disabled clients awaken to sexual feelings and often be surprised and delighted by it. It was time for me to apply this bit of wisdom to myself. So, I no longer had two sensitive breasts. I still had one, and a partner who never shied away from reimagining our life in the bedroom. And that was plenty.

∽

Scott was the first client I saw after returning to work, five months after my diagnosis. He was coping with an overriding fear that his penis was too small, and he had gone to drastic measures to enlarge it. A doctor had given him injections, which, instead of growing his penis, slightly misshaped it. The last thing he needed was my body image issues spilling over into our work together.

I held to my plan not to mention my mastectomy right away. From the outset, it had to be clear that he came first in our work together. When we undressed, I told him about my surgery, and invited him to feel my breasts. Scott cupped my right breast in his hand and lightly squeezed it. He did the same to the left. "The right one feels harder," he said. "Yup, they still haven't perfected reconstruction." Then we set about tackling his issues and the topic of my mastectomy didn't return.

Once again, I had learned the value of simple, straightforward communication and of appreciating the full breadth of sexuality. When a client finally comes to see a surrogate he is ready to work on himself, and a slightly lopsided bust has yet to prove a problem in my work.

In the third session with Scott, when it came time to do the mirror exercise, the new narrative of my breasts, which I had only begun to formulate, unveiled itself to me. As I looked at my reflection I said, simply, "I have had breast cancer, but was lucky that it was caught early. I had to have my right breast removed and reconstructed. Now it's not nearly as sensitive as my left. Even so, I like it to get equal attention."

℘

My practice continued to thrive, even though ordinary aging presented certain physical challenges. I was no longer as flexible or as nimble as I was when I first started as a surrogate. On the other hand, I had nearly four decades of experience to draw on and a level of expertise, sensitivity, and insight that I couldn't have had as a younger woman. My reputation in the field was established, and I had a coterie of therapists in the Bay Area, and even other parts of the country, who referred clients to me. Between my standing in the community and the dearth of surrogates, the work continued to roll in. In the wake of AIDS, surrogates left the practice in droves. I sometimes wonder how my profession would look today if the disease hadn't changed the course of it.

I could look back on a rich and rewarding career, and I was still in demand. In all of my years in this profession, my age has only been an issue for one client who referred to me as "no spring chicken." He and I actually wound up working well together after I explained to him that if he expected to be a hit with any woman, he should keep that kind of comment to himself—especially since he was hardly a young man himself.

Sometimes clients call me after our work is completed to get a confidence boost, or with questions that arise for them. They also often send me cards or emails thanking me or reflecting on our time together. In 1990, Mark O'Brien published the essay "On Seeing a Sex Surrogate" in *The Sun* magazine. He detailed how our work together unfolded in a way that only someone with his talents as a journalist and poet could have. I was moved by it, and so was Ben Lewin, a Los Angeles–based screenwriter and filmmaker.

In 2007, Ben visited me with an old friend of his who was also his chief financial backer. Like Mark, Ben had been afflicted with polio as a child and he walked with forearm crutches and a leg brace. I'm sure this was a primary reason Mark's story resonated so deeply with him. Between other projects, Ben started working on a screenplay based on Mark's article and our interview. He would send me drafts to review and check in occasionally, but long periods went by without any contact.

With Ben's busy schedule and the vagaries of the film world, it sometimes seemed that the project would languish. Then, in 2010, when I returned home from a trip to Boston to visit family, I found an oversized envelope in the stack of mail waiting for me on the dining room table. The screenplay was finished and it was tentatively titled *The Surrogate*.

From there an incredible cascade of good fortune began. The film received more financing and Ben secured three talented actors to appear in it. John Hawkes had been cast as Mark. I was thrilled. I had admired him in *Deadwood, Winter's Bone, The Perfect Storm*, and other movies, and I couldn't wait to see the chameleon-like actor turn into my erstwhile client. The inestimable William H. Macy was set to play Mark's priest and confidant. Several actresses were considered for the role of the surrogate.

When I learned who would be the onscreen version of me I was in my car. "Helen Hunt is going to play you." My heart sped up; I must have taken my foot off the gas because I soon realized my car was nearly at a stop. I was so stunned that I almost forgot I was driving. Pull over before you cause an accident, I thought and veered to the roadside. "Helen Hunt," I stammered into the cell phone. "That's right," said Ben. Academy Award–winning Helen Hunt, a bona fide star and a beautiful and respected actor, was going to play me. Was this really happening?

Ben also asked if I would serve as a consultant on the film, which would start shooting in May 2011. This would entail working with the two primary actors, and being on set for some of the filming. I made plans to fly to Los Angeles as soon as I got home.

~

I've always loved movies. Growing up in the '50s I went to our hometown theater almost every Saturday. That was before you could log on to the Internet or buy a book about filmmaking, so the workings of the Hollywood dream factory were opaque and mysterious to the general public. Even as an adult, I lost myself in onscreen magic, having little sense of what it took to create it. Being on the set with the cast and crew of the movie changed that. The amount of time, work, and energy that goes into a film is staggering. One thing I learned immediately is how much curiosity and thought underlies a great acting performance. Both Helen and John asked a number of smart questions about me, my work, and Mark. They honed in on the tiniest details and immersed themselves in the story.

Helen Hunt invited me to have lunch with her on one of the first days I was in Los Angeles. We met in Santa Monica, and as I sat at a table waiting, I saw her walk past the restaurant window, and, once again, felt like I was dreaming. Helen had so much genuine interest in me and my work that I quickly lost my anxiety about sitting across the table from an accomplished and celebrated actor. She taped much of our conversation and paid careful attention to the cadence and rhythm of my speech. The next day I went to her home and demonstrated Sensual Touch on her partner, who remained fully clothed.

By the time John Hawkes and I met, he had seen *Breathing Lessons*, an Academy Award–winning short documentary about Mark O'Brien, close to twenty times. One of the first things John said to me was how impressed and inspired he was by the courage Mark had shown throughout his life. He wanted his performance to honor him. John was in the process of reading every piece of Mark's writing he could get his hands on, and he had even learned how to type with a mouth stick, the way Mark had. I'll never forget the first time I saw John on set playing Mark. It was overwhelming. It was as if he had dissolved into Mark. As I sat there with my headphones listening to John deliver his lines in Mark's wheezy voice, I got chills.

Only one sadness shadowed this extraordinary time. Mark wouldn't be here to see the movie. In 1999, he succumbed to post-polio syndrome. I know he would have been tickled by the whole process, and I thought often about how he would have coached the filmmakers. One of the many things I love about the film is how Ben and John capture Mark's wit. If it's true that our spirits live on after death, I'm sure Mark is laughing at all the humor.

For a while, it seemed like every day something positive happened. In November 2011, I received an early Christmas gift when I learned that the film had been accepted to the Sundance Film Festival. It would debut on January 23, 2012. Not only that, but I was invited to attend the screening. I was heading to one of the most prestigious film festivals in the world.

I called my cousin and dear friend Susan, and she whooped so loud I had to pull the phone away from my ear. I set it down on an end table and switched to speaker mode before I asked if she wanted to join Bob and me in Utah.

The next day I hit some high-end thrift shops for something special to wear on the trip. I finally found a gorgeous beaded silk kimono-style top and pants to match. Where else had these clothes been worn? I wondered. I didn't know, but I couldn't imagine it had been to Sundance.

On the Saturday before the film was due to open, we arrived in Utah in the midst of a blizzard. The next morning we walked around the quaint Park City streets that were festooned with Sundance banners. They buzzed with excitement and the media was out in force. "The Sundance Film Festival" emblazoned the marquees of the theaters that dotted the downtown. CNN had requested an interview with me the day after the premiere.

I spent more time getting ready for the premiere than I had for any event in recent memory. I was anxious and excited. I had seen clips from the movie, but this was the first time I would view the finished product. It showed at the sprawling Eccles Theater, and when we arrived we were shunted off to an area designated for people involved with the film. Ben Lewin, Helen Hunt, John Hawkes, William H. Macy, and others from the cast and crew sat amid the packed house. As the film began, I squeezed Bob's hand. I still couldn't believe this was really happening.

The Surrogate was everything I could have hoped it would be. It was poignant, smart, beautifully acted, and funny. One of the things I loved the most about it was the thoughtful portrayal of my profession. I don't think it could have done a better job of revealing the complexities, challenges, and rewards of surrogacy work and the unique relationship that develops between surrogate and client. It was also one of the first times I had seen the sexuality of a disabled character handled with such honesty and grace. Maybe it's asking more than a movie can deliver, but I hope that disabled people will come away from it feeling that their sexuality has been affirmed and recognized, and reminded that they have as much of a right as anyone to explore and enjoy sex.

In our continuing string of luck, the film was sold to Fox Searchlight. It also won the special jury prize for ensemble acting and the audience award in the drama genre. I was touched by how many people wanted to meet me after the movie and how warmly they treated me. When I got back to the hotel, I called Jessica, who was only slightly less ecstatic about all of this than me. Hours later I was still wired, but I eventually slipped into sleep and out of the dream I had been living.

Back in Berkeley, I brushed off the stardust and returned to my work and life. So much had happened recently that I could never have imagined when I began as a surrogate. As a confused and frightened kid, I worried about a desolate future burdened with secrets and shame. I predicted a long string of doomed efforts to mold myself into inhuman standards that I was sure I was the only one who couldn't meet. As I look back, my life seems like a road with impossible twists and turns. I often wonder what it would be like today if I had been born in a different era, if I had never met Michael, if I had never heard of surrogacy. I know one thing for certain: The person I know as me wouldn't exist.

As I inch toward seventy, I appreciate more and more how much I have to be grateful for and how fortunate I've been. I was lucky to find a wonderful career and to be surrounded by so many smart, adventurous, caring people. My personal sexual revolution auspiciously paralleled our culture's, and in many ways was made possible by it. I am eternally grateful to the pioneers, rebels, and dreamers who made our society a little safer for women who embrace their sexuality. I have seen hundreds of clients, and I still can't think of anything I would rather do with my life than to help people more fully express and enjoy their sexuality. Confusion about sex remains rampant in our culture. An all-pervasive media promulgates misconceptions, distortions, and falsehood about it, while retrograde political forces continue to threaten sexual education and freedom. I know that the men and women with whom I've worked are but a small fraction of the people who struggle with their sexuality. Still, I feel gratified when I look back at my career and recall how I helped my clients build healthier, happier sex lives.

That I am encircled by a loving, supportive family means that I am doubly gifted with happiness in both my work and personal life. Bob and I have shared nearly half of our lives. It was with him that I learned that love wasn't something I had to earn anew each day. It could be received and given unconditionally. A loving partnership transforms the individuals in it into better people than they would be on their own. It both uplifts and grounds a life. It is only because of Bob that I know this, and my love for him is immeasurable. Today my children are successful, confident, and caring adults. Michael and I gave them a childhood full of love and support, encouragement, and guidance. Together we laid the ground for them to become the people they are today. This is the only accomplishment I take more pride in than my surrogacy career.

I'm more in demand than ever from the media, and I still get asked to explain how I'm different from a prostitute. As I watched *The Sessions*, as the film was later retitled, I wondered if it would make the difference clear to the general public. If it doesn't, I'm not worried. I can think of worse things to be conflated with, and what separates surrogates from prostitutes is significant. When people have difficulty grasping it, I turn to my beloved and late friend Steven Brown's cooking analogy that I've so often relied on to help me through that question: Seeing a prostitute is like going to a restaurant. Seeing a surrogate is like going to culinary school. I'm sixty-eight now, and I have no intention of hanging up my apron.

recommended resources

books

Better Than I Ever Expected: Straight Talk about Sex after Sixty, Joan Price, Oakland, California, Seal Press, 2005.

Changing Bodies, Changing Lives: A Book for Teens on Sex and Relationships, Ruth Bell Alexander, New York City, Three Rivers Press, 1998.

Cockfidence: The Extraordinary Lover's Guide to Being the Man You Want to Be and Driving Women Wild, Celeste Hirschman, MA and Danielle Harel, Ph.D., Somatica Press, 2011.

The Dance of Anger: A Woman's Guide to Changing the Patterns of Intimate Relationships, Harriet Lerner, Ph.D., New York City, Perennial Currents, 2005.

Erotic Massage, Kenneth Ray Stubbs, Ph.D., New York City, Tarcher, 1999

The Erotic Mind: Unlocking the Inner Sources of Sexual Passion and Fulfillment, Jack Morin, Ph.D., New York City, Harper Perennial, 1996.

Femalia, Joani Blank, San Francisco, California, Last Gasp Press, 2011.

For Each Other: Sharing Sexual Intimacy, Lonnie Barbach Ph.D., New York City, Anchor, 1983.

For Yourself: The Fulfillment of Female Sexuality, Lonnie Barbach, Ph.D., New York City, Signet, 2000.

Getting the Love You Want: A Guide for Couples, Harville Hendrix, Ph.D., New York City, Henry Holt & Co, 2007.

A Guide to Getting It On, Paul Joannides and Daerick Gross, Waldport, Oregon, Goofy Foot Press, 2000.

Keeping the Love You Find: A Personal Guide, Harville Hendrix, Ph.D., New York City, Atria Books, 1993.

Mating in Captivity: Unlocking Erotic Intelligence, Esther Perel, New York City, Harper Perennial, 2007.

My Body, My Self for Boys, Lynda Madaras and Area Madaras, New York City, William Morrow Paperbacks, 2007

My Body, My Self for Girls, Lynda Madaras and Area Madaras, New York City, William Morrow Paperbacks, 2007.

Naked at Our Age: Talking Out Loud about Senior Sex, Joan Price, Oakland, California, Seal Press, 2011.

The New Male Sexuality: The Truth about Men, Sex, and Pleasure, Bernie Zilbergeld, Ph.D., New York City, Bantam, 1999.

A New View of a Woman's Body: A Fully Illustrated Guide, the Federation of Feminist Women's Health Centers, Illustrations by Suzann Gage, L. Ac. RNC, NP, San Diego, California, Feminist Health Press, 1991.

Petals, Nick Karras, San Diego, California, Crystal River Publishing, 2003.

Resurrecting Sex: Solving Sexual Problems and Revolutionizing Your Relationship, David Schnarch, Ph.D., New York City, Harper Perennial, 2003

Romantic Interludes: A Sensuous Lovers Guide, Kenneth Ray Stubbs, Ph.D., with Louise-André Saulnier, Tucson, Arizona, Secret Garden Press, 1996

Sex for One: The Joy of Selfloving, Betty Dodson, Ph.D., New York City, Three Rivers Press, 1996.

Women's Sexualities: Generations of Women Share Intimate Secrets of Sexual Self-Acceptance, Carol Rinkleib Ellison, Ph.D., Oakland, California, New Harbinger Publications, 2006.

sex and disability

Enabling Romance: A Guide to Love, Sex, and Relationships for People with Disabilities (and the People Who Care About Them), Ken Kroll and Erica Levy Klein, Horsham, Pennsylvania, No Limits Communications, 2001.

Not Made of Stone: The Sexual Problems of Handicapped People, K. Heslinga, Thomas 1974.

The Sensuous Wheeler: Sexual Adjustment for the Spinal Cord Injured, Barry J. Rabin, Ph.D., Multi Media Resource Center, 1980.

Sex and Back Pain: Advice on Restoring Comfortable Sex Lost to Back Pain, Lauren Andrew Hebert, PT, Greenville, Maine, Impacc USA, 1997.

Sex When You're Sick: Reclaiming Sexual Health after Illness or Injury, Anne Katz, Santa Barbara, California, Praeger, 2009.

Sex-Role Issues in Mental Health, Kay F. Schaffer, Addison-Wesley Publishers, 1980.

Sexual Options for Paraplegics and Quadriplegics, Thomas O. Mooney, Theodore M. Cole, M.D., and Richard Chilgren, M.D., New York City, Little Brown & Co., 1975.

Sexuality after Spinal Cord Injury: Answers to Your Questions, Stanley H. DuCharme and Kathleen M. Gill, Baltimore, Maryland, Brookes Publishing Company, 1996.

The Ultimate Guide to Sex and Disability: For All of Us Who Live with Disabilities, Chronic Pain, and Illness, Miriam Kaufman, Fran Odette, and Cory Silverberg, Berkeley, California, Cleis Press, 2007.

videos, toys, etc.

Betty Dodson, Ph.D.
dodsonandross.com

Good Vibrations
goodvibes.com

Kenneth Ray Stubbs
secretgardenpublishing.com

sex information

San Francisco Sex Information
sfsi.org

Sexuality Information and Education Council of the United States
siecus.org

acknowledgments

Writing a book is always a team effort. It was our good fortune to be part of a team of stellar professionals, without whom *An Intimate Life* would have remained a dream. Cheryl and Lorna wish to thank Charlie Winton, Liz Parker, Maren Fox, Kelly Winton, Jodi Hammerwold, and the rest of the staff at Counterpoint for all of their hard work and dedication to this project. Brooke Warner, our editor, deserves much credit for making this book readable, lively, and professional. Thanks are also due to Brad Bunnin, our publishing consultant, who provided us with invaluable guidance. Finally, our profound gratitude goes to David Cole for bringing us together.

From Cheryl: I want to thank my Nanna Fournier for her unconditional love. My mother, for understanding that mothers and daughters can also be friends. My father, for his wonderful sense of humor, something that is necessary for a fulfilled life. My children, who are the absolute loves of my life. All my dear nonjudgmental friends who have given me support throughout the years. My husband, Bob, who taught me how to accept unconditional love. Michael Paul Cohen, without whom I would never have moved to California and discovered the work that has so profoundly affected my life. And Lorna Garano, who understood my stories and masterfully helped transcribe them onto the written page. My appreciation is eternal.

From Lorna: I would like to thank my family for their unending support and unconditional love. I also wish to express my gratitude to my coauthor, Cheryl Cohen Greene. It was an honor to help her write her story and to bring her wise, compassionate, and generous spirit to life in these pages. Last, but not least, my heartfelt thanks go to my partner, Peter Handel, the love of my life.

about the authors

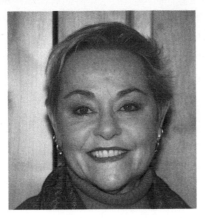

CHERYL T. COHEN GREENE, DHS, has been in private clinical practice as a surrogate partner and consultant in human sexuality since 1973. She was trained in the Masters and Johnson modality and was on the training staff of San Francisco Sex Information for nineteen years. She is a certified sex educator and clinical sexologist, and in 2004 earned her DHS (Doctor of Human Sexuality) from the Institute for the Advanced Study of Human Sexuality in San Francisco. Currently, Cohen Greene serves as the vice president of IPSA (International Professional Surrogates Association), and was one of the founders of BASA (Bay Area Surrogates Association), a support group for surrogate partners in the San Francisco Bay Area.

Cohen Greene lectures widely and she is frequently sought out by national media. She has been interviewed by CNN, *Larry King Live*, *San Francisco Chronicle*, *Cosmopolitan*, *Men's Health*, and other national outlets. Visit her at **www.cherylcohengreene.com**

LORNA GARANO is a freelance writer and publicist based in the San Francisco Bay Area. Visit her at **www.lornagarano.com**